CHI KUNG—ENERGY FOR LIFE

Contributors to this book:

Linda Chase Broda
Jesse Dammann
Russell DesMarais
Ron Diana
Bill Douglas
John Du Cane
Gaspar Garcia
Garri Garripoli
Roger Jahnke
Damaris Jarboux
Jerry Alan Johnson
Mark Johnson
Marcia Kerwit
Richard Leirer
Dennis Lewis
Adrian Lowe
Tina Marrow Rasheed
Ronnie Robinson
Ken Sancier
Solala Towler
Gunther Weil
Michael Winn

JAMES MACRITCHIE

Chi Kung

Energy for Life

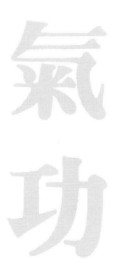

Thorsons

Thorsons
An Imprint of HarperCollins*Publishers*
77–85 Fulham Palace Road
Hammersmith, London W6 8JB

The Thorsons website address is:
www.thorsons.com

and *Thorsons*
are trademarks of HarperCollins*Publishers* Limited

Published by Thorsons 2002

10 9 8 7 6 5 4 3 2 1

Text © James MacRitchie, 2002

James MacRitchie asserts the moral right to
be identified as the author of this work

A catalogue record for this book
is available from the British Library

ISBN 0-00-714568-3

Printed and bound in Great Britain by
Scotprint, Haddington, Scotland

Photography by Robin Matthews
Illustrations by PCA, and Jennie Dooge

Note from the Publisher

*Any information given in this book is not intended to be taken as a replacement for medical
advice. Any person with a condition requiring medical attention should consult a qualified
practitioner or therapist.*

Contents

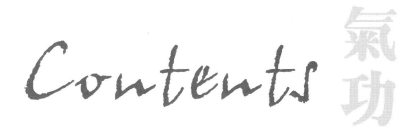

This book is dedicated to the
National Qigong (Chi Kung) Association * USA,
my brothers and sisters in The Tao.

Acknowledgments 氣功

I would foremost like to thank my wonderful wife and partner, Damaris Jarboux, and my children Sonnet, Hagan, and John for being who they are. My love beyond words to my late mother Joan Frederica Tilley (pictured on page 174 after walking to the top of Moel Famau, in North Wales, UK, in her 82nd year), my sister Susan, brother Malcolm, and all of my extended family.

The folks at HarperCollins for bringing this book about: Belinda Budge, Wanda Whiteley, Paul Redhead, Samantha Grant, Jo Ridgeway, Kate Latham, and to Matthew Cory, my editor, who made all of the words work. To Robin Matthews and Aitken for the photography. To the models, for their Chi: Mark Nash, Judith Frances Solomons and Vicki Maschio, and to Dan Docherty for invaluable production assistance.

To the 22 contributors, listed at the end of the book, who added so much.

For insights and editorial with ideas and text: John Churchill, Peter Conti, Jesse Dammann, Deborah Dodds, John Firor, Finney Fox-Davis, Jennifer Hoyt, Judy Jacobsen, Barbara Jones, Marion Parker, Rachel Rodgers, and Beth Sims. To Carla Gholson for editorial guidance and feedback. To Prof. Fang, Ting-yu, and Ms. Hua, Yuan at WASMQ. To my valued friends, for all and everything: Julie Carpenter, Robert Carpenter, Bill Harpe, Robert B. McFarland, Richard Ruster, David Scott, Robert Schuman, and Eddie and Debbie Shapiro. And to Anna Wise for all we shared and share.

With special fond remembrance and appreciation of the late Danny Connor of Manchester, a Chi Kung pioneer and an example for us all. Good one, Danny.

To my teachers, students, professional colleagues, and friends too numerous to mention individually. Special acknowledgment to Master Mantak Chia and Prof. J.R. Worsley.

And thanks to Prof. Jin Huai Wang for his calligraphy of The Tao.

And finally, to you, the reader—the purpose for doing this book. I hope that it helps spark in you what it did in me. To all, my great appreciation and thanks.

Jim

Preface

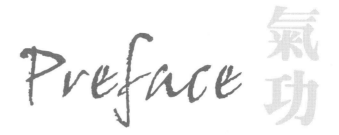

Just what is this marvelous practice called Chi Kung? What are we doing when we do Chi Kung? In a sense, we are stepping out of our mundane, limited sense of reality and opening ourselves up to a richer, wider, and deeper form of experience. We are allowing what is infinite to be contained by what is so finite—our own bodies. Our own energy system is a microcosm of the very planets and stars turning gently in space. Our own minds grow in breadth to contain the universe. Our very own sense of ourself expands into a greater, richer sense of divine self—or what the Chinese call Wuji, the primordial origin of all life.

When we do our practice—our form, our breathing, our visualizations, our movements —we align ourselves with our own origin, our divine birthright. We are allowing ourselves to become "empty vessels," ready to be filled with the energy of the universe itself. As all the sages down through history tell us: we, in our humble and often confused states of being, are still a part of the whole, a piece of the totality of it all. What better way to experience that consciously than to practice Chi Kung? What better way to step forth into new dimensions of experience and knowledge? What better opportunity to allow ourselves the freedom, the strength, the deepness of character and intelligence to begin to let go of the chains of illusion and limitation that we have been told we are? We are ever and always so much more than that!

When we do Chi Kung we are saying "yes" to miracles and an openness to change, healing, and growth. We are taking the first of a thousand steps into the unknown, into the very Tao itself. We are, at the very least, allowing ourselves to heal, to grow, to change along with the great changing that is always and constant. We are aligning ourselves with the great cycles of change and, in doing so, freeing ourselves from the tyranny of time and the limitations of life. We are setting ourselves free so that we can soar like the butterfly, and flow like the water that was so beloved by the ancient Taoist sages. In the end, we are practiced by our Chi Kung as much as we practice it. One breath at a time, one movement at a time, one moment at a time.

Solala Towler

Introduction

氣功

After a long history of being held secret in the East, Chi Kung is at last becoming widely known in the West, and people are becoming aware of its profound benefits and effects. Most people are concerned about their energy, that mysterious and elusive aspect of ourselves that fuels us, and gives us the health, strength, stamina, optimism, and spirit that is the foundation of everything else in our lives. Chi Kung is a way to work with, develop, and cultivate our own personal Energy, which is the very essence of the Life inside us.

Chi Kung ("energy cultivation") encompasses the whole range of our lives, from normal everyday activities, such as sitting and walking, to the exploration of the deepest levels of soul and spirit. It is based upon the principles of The Tao—the ancient Chinese philosophy also known as The Way of Nature.

This book is a complete guide to Chi Kung. It contains not only a comprehensive overview of Chi Kung theory and practice, but also contributions from 22 leading Western teachers and practitioners, providing a unique insight into this powerful Oriental discipline.

The entry of Chi Kung and the broader field of Chinese Medicine into the West over the last 50 years has not been without its problems. Not least of these has been the difficulty in translating the terms used by one culture into another. The name "Chi Kung" was chosen in 1954 by a Chinese Communist Government sub-committee as a name for the enormous range of energy practices that had been developed in China over the course of its history. When the Chinese Government later revised their language from ideographic (calligraphy) to phonetic (Western alphabet), the spelling changed to "Qigong." Other spellings include

"Chee Gung" and "Ji Kong." In this book the spelling Chi Kung was chosen partly because it is widely familiar through T'ai Chi and Acupuncture.

Indeed, Acupuncture, now firmly established and widely accepted in the West, is itself considered by many to be a form of Chi Kung—a way of "working with energy." Chi Kung uses the same energy pathways, points, principles, and charts as Acupuncture. However, the word "Acupuncture" is not Chinese; in fact, it is said to have been coined by a Jesuit priest serving in Asia in the 1500s, when he saw this practice being performed. The Chinese call it "Zhen Jou" (Needle and Heat). I now call my professional practice Zhen Jou Chi Kung, in respect to its origins.

In the 1950s the Chinese Government undertook the amalgamation of the whole field of Chinese Medicine in order to bring it into line with Western Medicine. The result of this process was named Traditional Chinese Medicine (TCM), although the "traditional" element of this term is misleading. TCM comprehensively describes the mechanics of the energy system, but it specifically casts aside the traditional aspects such as Taoist and Buddhist philosophy, the emotions, poetry, and spirit. In the Chi Kung that you will read about in this book, the traditional aspects of its foundation have been restored.

HOW TO USE THIS BOOK

This book is divided into five parts:

Part One	**What Is Chi Kung?**
Part Two	**Your Energy System**
Part Three	**Activating Your Energy**
Part Four	**More Chi, More Life**
Part Five	**Everyday Chi Kung**

Part One gives an overview of Chi Kung, describing its origins and history, the different forms of Chi Kung that are available, and the immense benefits that each form of Chi Kung may bring to each of us. Present day scientific research into body energy is also discussed.

Part Two describes the structure and function of the body's energy system, to explain what it is and how it works. An understanding of this is essential before one can go on to learn to control and use it. By way of comparison, other Eastern and Western energy systems are also presented.

Part Three examines the attitude and preparation needed before embarking on any Chi Kung practice. This is followed by a series of beginning practices that will provide anyone with a foundation for good energy health.

Part Four moves on to a higher level and contains many contributions from respected authorities in the field. These include advanced practices that you can use for yourself, your family, friends, students, and clients. There is also a survey of the Clinical Chi Kung treatments and techniques that you are most likely to encounter in the West.

Finally, Part Five describes the relevance of Chi Kung to the normal activities of ordinary life, and shows how you can apply the principles and practices of Chi Kung to getting the best out of everyday living. It shows how it relates to waking, working, resting, and sleeping, as well as to children, schools, the elderly, and those with special needs. The book ends with a look at Chi Kung's relevance to the global society.

By practicing Chi Kung you will be able to gain control and mastery of your own energy, and embody your Chi. There is no better thing that you could do for yourself. My wish is that this book serves to guide you on the Way.

James MacRitchie
Boulder, Colorado
June 2002

PART ONE

What Is Chi Kung?

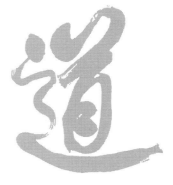

CHAPTER ONE

Introducing Chi Kung

氣功

Chi Kung is a miraculous, mysterious, and wonderful thing. It covers a vast territory and is in many ways the missing piece of Western culture. It can be compared to music, or dance, in that just as there are many kinds of these, with all manner of applications, so there are many kinds of Chi Kung.

As is widely known, "Chi" means "Energy," but "Kung" is a term for which there is no easy equivalent in the West, yet it is at the foundation of much Chinese medical and spiritual practice. "Kung" probably best translates into the word "Cultivation." So, through practicing Chi Kung you practice Energy Cultivation.

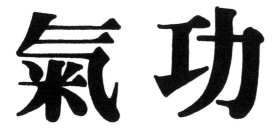

4 THE FORMS OF CHI KUNG

There are many ancient forms of Chi Kung that have been faithfully transmitted down through the generations, and there are new forms that are being developed at the present time. There are special styles that are family secrets, only passed down through the male lineage, and there are traditional forms such "The Five Animal Frolics" and "The Six Healing Sounds" that have been elaborated, changed, and expanded almost beyond recognition, until it seems that everyone has their own version.

Everyone has their own individual style, but as when traveling by different routes to reach the same destination, they mostly arrive at the same place in the end! One consequence of this is that there are no agreed standards—there is no more a "right" way to do Chi Kung than there is a "right" way to dance. There do, however, remain some common characteristics that all forms of Chi Kung share.

COMMON CHARACTERISTICS OF CHI KUNG

Internal and External
This is a basic division into two broad categories. All Chi Kung involves movement and/or stillness. Internal Chi Kung, which requires stillness, is called Nei Dan. External Chi Kung, which involves movement, is called Wei Dan. These are also respectively known as the "static arts" and the "dynamic arts." They can also be combined.

Posture, Breathing, and Mind
All forms of Chi Kung use a combination of these three basic components.

The Meridian system and the Energy points
All Chi Kung is based on the energy anatomy of the Meridian system and the Energy points.

The Three Tan T'ien
These are the three important areas in the lower, middle, and upper body (*see* page 83), which are considered to be major centers of energy.

Organs and Tissues
All forms of Chi Kung affect and cultivate the organs, tissues, and functions of the body.

Nei Dan and Wei Dan are the two fundamental categorizations of Chi Kung, and they can be combined and integrated in many ways. It is also possible to know a great deal about one without knowing anything about the other.

Internal Chi Kung

Internal Chi Kung (Nei Dan) includes all kinds of exercises that do not involve any external movement. The mind is fully conscious during these exercises. Some of them can be seen as meditation, and these include categories of practice such as Relaxing Exercises, Breathing Exercises, and Standing Exercises. These practices change the body's functions from a state of energy consuming to one of energy restoring, and they contribute to the body's ability to self-regulate, self-repair, and self-regenerate. In Nei Dan exercises, specific Posture, Breathing, and Mind methods are used to control and direct the Chi.

- Posture. There are three basic variations of posture—standing, sitting, and lying.
- Breathing. Breathing practice is a very precise and important aspect of Chi Kung. It brings into the body one of the three components of the body's energy—Oxygen, the energy from Heaven (the others are Food, the energy of Earth, and the inherited energy of Yuan Chi in the kidneys, an aspect of Jing).
- Mind. The mind has the ability to direct the Chi in the body, and there are four major methods for doing this:
  - focusing on certain energy points;
  - focusing on beautiful and peaceful scenes or images;
  - focusing on a particular idea, person, or memory;
  - focusing on the meaning of words (such as Relaxation, Tranquility, and Peace).

There is a wide variety of ways to combine the techniques of Posture, Breathing, and Mind. These include Relaxing exercises to prepare and warm-up, and Quiescent Chi Kung to calm the mind; Breathing exercises using particular postures and patterns of breathing; Standing exercises which can be accompanied by variations of hand positions which create geometric patterns of the meridian system that serve to drive the energy in a particular direction.

External Chi Kung

External Chi Kung (Wei Dan) refers to all the forms and styles involving external movement. There are a very large number of these exercises, sets, forms, and sequences:

- Classic forms, passed down through history, which have undergone innumerable permutations, variations, and adaptations;

- Sets of exercises used for treating specific symptoms and conditions. These can comprise a form of Medical Chi Kung;
- Sequences designed to cultivate physical fitness and strength, as in "Hard" Chi Kung and martial arts training;
- Long-standing family secrets and traditions;
- Forms recently developed by doctors and practitioners;
- Procedures that are spiritually transforming;
- Exercises which are useful when getting up in the morning, comparable to doing stretches.

Some of these exercises are easy to learn and do. Some are very hard and take a lot of time, patience, and practice—if, indeed, you can find somebody willing to teach you. Some are so esoteric, refined, and difficult that you would only be taught them in a monastic setting, and only after you had proven yourself worthy to receive such teachings. Many of the moving sequences are extraordinarily graceful and beautiful to watch.

As with other skills, the more you practice external Chi Kung the more proficient you become. Learning a particular form embodies it in your being and it becomes part of you—part of the way you move and experience yourself. It is truly an investment in yourself.

CHI KUNG AND OTHER PRACTICES

There are specific characteristics that distinguish external Chi Kung from other kinds of physical exercises such as aerobics, sports training, and ballet.

- It uses a comprehensive knowledge of the body's Chi and meridian system.
- It is based upon the theories of Oriental anatomy and physiology.
- It is practiced in an inward state of peace, achieved through specific postures, breathing, and mental focusing.
- It requires calming the spirit and regulating Chi in very particular ways.

The Benefits of Chi Kung

There are many positive reasons for taking on the significant commitment of studying and practicing Chi Kung, but the very simplest is "because it makes you feel good," and this can mean feeling health, well-being, emotional clarity and balance, integration, sensitivity, clear-mindedness, happiness, and satisfaction. It is also a way of developing spiritually and accessing your higher self. To one degree or another these can all be achieved, or improved, through Chi Kung.

This may be experienced with subjective sensations such as feeling bright-eyed, clear-headed, high-spirited, euphoric, at perfect peace, completely relaxed, or deeply refreshed. Or it may be purely in physical terms, such as increased stamina, better digestion, improved circulation, increased resistance to illness, and decreased tiredness and fatigue.

Chi Kung may also serve to eliminate specific problems and symptoms. In China, it is said that Chi Kung can be used for:

- **Curing illness;**
- **Prevention of disease;**
- **Strengthening the constitution;**
- **Avoiding premature ageing;**
- **Prolonging life.**

In addition, there are other potential benefits, such as gaining personal power, developing extraordinary abilities, entering into heightened states of consciousness, and living in bliss.

The Origins and History of Chi Kung

Before looking at the practice of Chi Kung in more detail, it is useful to step back and look at it from a historical and cultural perspective. The best place to start is with a short history of China.

THE HISTORY OF CHINA

Prior to 221BC the land we now know as China was divided into many separate areas which were ruled by different dynasties. There is reported to have been a legendary kingdom called Hsia as far back as 2000BC From approximately 1000BC–221BC there was a Feudal age, which ended with the 250 years of the so-called Warring States period.

In 246BC, a young man named Chao Cheng ascended to the throne of one of the smaller states. By 221BC he had progressively conquered all of the other states and created one country, in a manner comparable to Alexander the Great. He used his family name along with the name of one of the great legendary Emperors, and called himself Chhin Shih Huang Ti, The First Emperor of Chhin. As well as unifying the country for the first time, he disbanded the ancient feudal system, created a common civil code, and established one written language. His rule was draconian, but it lasted for only 14 years, although his influence was so great that the family name of Chhin became the basis for the name of the land and its people.

During this era, comparable to the Golden Age of ancient Greece, some of the most profound and enlightened thinkers of China's history appeared, who determined and still underlie and influence its culture. These included Lao Tzu, Chuang Tzu, Lieh Tzu, and K'ung Fu-tzu (Confucius). Tzu simply means Master. Some of the most important and influential books were written at this time, including *The I Ching* (*The Book of Changes*—considered to be the oldest existing book), *The Nei Ching* (*The Classic of Internal Medicine*), and *The Tao Te Ching* (*The Book of The Way and its Virtue*). The authors of many of these classics are unknown as are the exact dates of their writing or compilation—like the Bible, their origins are lost in legend and pre-history.

After the death of the first Emperor the history of China progressed in a yo-yo fashion over the next thousand years or so. First it would be unified, then it would break apart into separate feudal states, only to be unified again by a determined Emperor.

The First Partition	**AD 221–AD 265**
The Second Unification	**AD 265–AD 479**
The Second Partition	**AD 479–AD 581**
The Third Unification	**AD 581–AD 906**
The Third Partition	**AD 907–AD 1227**

For the last 1,000 years or so China has been unified, although under different dynasties. Having been isolated previously from most outside influences, at the end of the 19th century China was opened up to the Western world, and this influenced its efforts to modernize. After World War II, the Communists gained power, and they imposed strict controls on information and education in much the same way as the dynasties of earlier times.

One of the most important differences between how we have come to view the world in the West and how the Chinese look at it, is that while their view of life is organized around, and based on, an understanding of energy, ours is based on a mastery of material objects. The implications of this are enormous, particularly in the difference between East and West in understanding just what a human being is. This difference is the reason that we have no equivalent to Chi Kung. To appreciate this, we need to look in more detail at the history of Taoism.

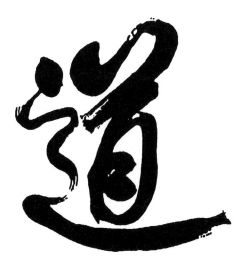

The Tao

Taoism is the major tradition at the root of Chi Kung. In China there was a wide range of religious and spiritual movements, and over the course of history different schools grew, developed, flourished, and declined. There were the Confucians, the Naturalists, the Buddhists, the Mohists, the Logicians, the Legalists, and many others, but by far the most influential and relevant group in relation to Chi Kung were the Taoists.

Taoism is a natural philosophy. It is based on observation of, and alignment with, the natural and organic order of things—from planetary movements and the progression of the seasons, to our individual feelings and how they function. Taoists can be thought of as early scientists, in that they observed nature, understood its ways, and aspired to act in accord with it. Today in China, Taoism is still very much alive, adapting to the conditions and circumstances of the times.

Lao Tzu and The Tao Te Ching

The name Tao is taken from the book *The Tao Te Ching*, attributed to Lao Tzu (a name which means Old Master), and it is supposed to have been written in the fifth century BC. In general terms, the word "Tao" can be translated as Way, Path, or Road, "Te" means Virtue, and "Ching" means Book or Classic—so, *Tao Te Ching* can be translated as "*The Book of the Way and its Virtue.*"

The Tao Te Ching is a collection of insights, wisdom, and teachings. It contains pieces of text, such as proverbs, strung together without any real connection or meaning between them. The text explores the issues of knowledge, time, language and meaning, and "The Way." It uses paradox to force us to rethink. The Tao is beyond the ability of language to describe. It is a state of consciousness and an attitude toward living and life.

Chuang Tzu and Lieh Tzu

Two other major figures of Taoism were Chuang Tzu and Lieh Tzu. Chuang Tzu lived in the reigns of King Hui and King Hsuan of Ch'i during the Warring States period, 370–301BC. He viewed a sage as a recluse who rejected power, authority, and position as being illusionary and dangerous. He was concerned with freeing the mind from conventional ideas and patterns of behavior, in order to see deeper into the nature of things. For him, this way leads to freedom.

Lieh Tzu was revered by Chuang Tzu as a sage. He is said to have lived in the wilds, far removed from the world. The book which bears his name, from the second and third century BC, is a collection of stories, jokes, tales, practical tricks, legends, reflections, and musings. To Lieh Tzu, the Tao is understood as the origin and purpose of life; it is immanent and all pervading.

THE CHARACTERISTICS OF TAOISM

While there were many other Taoist teachers, some of the essential characteristics of Taoism can be summarized as follows:

1 There is a basic concern with social welfare.
2 There was a preoccupation with religious mysticism.
3 Much emphasis was placed on the training of the individual for Immortality (see page 22).
4 The foundation of scientific attitude was established, with a concern for the observation of nature. There was a consciousness of the nature of change and transformation—the Taoists distrusted logic and reason. For the Taoists, Nature is the mother of all things.

THE BASIC PRINCIPLES OF TAOISM

Wu Wei. This is best described as non-action or non-interference. Wu Wei is the art of being in Harmony with the Tao, so that everything happens as it should, of its own accord.

Change. Change is the essence of The Way. We all know that everything changes, but there is an underlying principle for this change. These principles are exemplified in the great classic of Chinese thought, The *I Ching—The Book of Changes*.

The Water Way. The principles of Transformation, Relativity, Yieldingness, and the Feminine Principle have been described together as The Water Way. Water is a primary symbol for

Taoists—it flows on, it fills all the open spaces, it is unstoppable, and it always finds the easiest route.

Some Taoists also believe in magic, the existence of realms of nature not perceivable to ordinary consciousness, in similar terms to shamanism, and in the Hsien, perfected immortals who live in the immortal realm.

To the Taoists, the Tao is the primary ground of everything. This basic credo is reflected in Chapter 42 of the *Tao Te Ching*:

> *The Tao is the origin of the One,*
> *The One created the two,*
> *The two formed the three.*
> *From the three came forth all life.*

This means that from Tao comes the origin; from the origin comes Yin and Yang; from Yin and Yang comes Heaven, Earth, and Humanity; and from these, all forms of existence.

"PURE" TAOISM AND FOLK TAOISM

Folk Taoism is a religion and a faith of the ordinary people, and various schools and traditions developed over the years with their own temples and priests. It was not for 300 years that Taoism came to be named after Lao Tzu, and by this time it had incorporated many of the folk beliefs and much of the religion of the ordinary people. In Folk Taoism there are legendary, saint-like figures, The Eight Immortals, who embody what might be seen as the basic archetypes of human nature. These were the characters who the common people of China—the farmers, merchants, tradesmen, and laborers—believed, and believe, in. There is a Taoist "Pope" and a Taoist Hell—the destination for anybody who transgressed the established morality and virtues. There is also a Taoist canon, a collection of essential scriptures on every aspect of life—from spiritual training, to divination, astrology, performing marriages, and burying the dead. One significant attitude is embodied in a belief in the importance of the individual self, rather than staying bound to Filial Piety and Ancestor Worship, in which each person was compelled to see themselves simply as a link in a chain of family continuity.

Above all else, there was one thing that all Taoists aspired to, a goal to achieve and be measured by, and this was to "Attain The Tao"—to achieve the state of being in which one understood, embodied, and lived in the Tao, the Way.

Buddhist Chi Kung

When speaking of Buddhist Chi Kung we refer to the Chi Kung based on the teachings of Shakyamuni Buddha. In general terms, this emphasizes the control and cultivation of Mind, the elimination of desires, and compassion for all living creatures. Interest is also laid on Wisdom and Illumination.

However, there is one other figure of utmost importance who must also be mentioned—Bodhidharma (P'u T'i Ta Mo, as he is known in China), the founder of Ch'an (Zen) Buddhism. Ta Mo created two sets of exercises—"The Muscle Change and Bone Marrow Washing" classic, and "The Hands of the Eighteen Luohans."

The Origins of the Hands of the Eighteen Luohans

It is said that in the year AD527, an Indian monk named Ta Mo came to the Shaolin monastery in the Songshan mountains of Hanan province to spread the teachings of the Buddha. He sat and faced the wall of his cave retreat for nine years, meditating in silence to seek enlightenment. During these years of meditation, Ta Mo found that the cumulative effects of not moving his body and limbs for a long time, together with the bitter cold and wind around his mountain retreat, caused him fatigue, aches, and pains. His disciples also suffered these ailments and often dozed off during meditation. To combat these hazards, as well as keeping them all fit and strong enough to defend themselves against bandits and wild beasts, Ta Mo put together a set of exercises based partly on Buddhist yoga, partly on existing fitness arts, and partly on his observations of animal behavior. The exercises he passed down were known as the Hands of the Eighteen Luohans.

During the Yuan Dynasty (1264–1368), the Hands of the Eighteen Luohans (consisting of 18 movements) was further enlarged to 72 movements, and later still to 179, forming the basis of Shaolin Chuan-Fa (Kung Fu), which went on to influence the development of all branches of Oriental fighting arts. These movements were passed down from generation to generation in the Shaolin Temple.

The Hands of the Eighteen Luohans work at all levels of the human being—physical, mental, and spiritual. Physically, they are a set of rigorous exercises that stretch and strengthen the body—the bones, muscles, tendons, and joints. They also drain the channels and improve the circulation of blood and energy, and they achieve this by working with the polarity of Yin/Yang in the movements. Deep abdominal breathing oxygenates the organism, bringing in a surplus of energy that is transmuted into a higher consciousness.

True to their origin, the Hands of the Eighteen Luohans follow and comply with Buddhist principles, and are an indispensable exercise for anybody who practices sitting meditation or wants to keep fit. When Bodhidharma created these movements, he sought an exercise that would train the body and mind to bring the Soul closer to Truth.

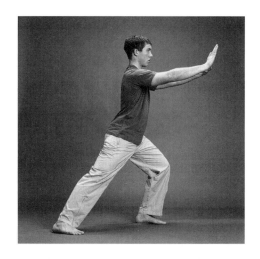

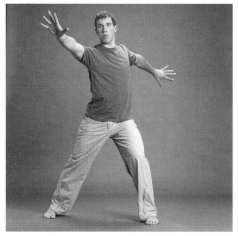

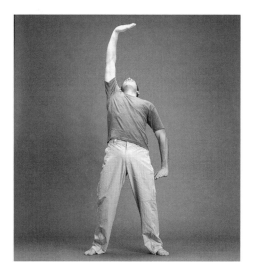

CHAPTER TWO

Energy and Life

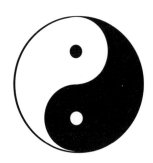

A Language of Energy

Energy is Life, but, remarkably, a language of Energy does not exist in the West. Language gives us both a means of expressing meaning, experience, and sensation, and a way of understanding these things ourselves. So, without a language of Energy, to a degree we are deprived of a conscious awareness of our own lives. It is fortunate that the human organism has an inbuilt ability to run its own energy system, but in order to develop our understanding and self-expression it is important to be aware of the four major components of the energy system in Chi Kung. These are:

1 Yin and Yang;

2 The Five Elements;

3 The Percentage Scale;

4 Volume Control.

Yin and Yang represent the polar opposites in any given situation, just as we know something by comparing it to something else—hot and cold, full and empty, still and moving, expanding and contracting, above and below, up and down, right and left, and front and back. Our experience is defined by these polarities, and thinking in these terms provides a method of describing experience.

The Five Elements (or Five Phases) are a means of describing the basic irreducible quality of something. Each of the Five Elements has corresponding organs, temperature, color, and direction. This allows us to describe an internal temperature as hot, cold, warm, cool, or mild; an internal color as green, red, yellow, white, or blue; an indication of location as up, down, right, left, or center. The language of the Five Elements is the language of our own internal structure.

The Percentage Scale is not usually identified as an internal mechanism, but it underlies everything we do. We have an inherent means of weighing one thing against another in percentage terms, and it happens automatically and intuitively. For instance, this is how we know the relative amount of effort we need to exert when picking up an empty cup as opposed to an ingot of lead. Similarly, we can divide our attention into parts, for instance, 50 percent to each hand or 25 percent to each hand and foot. Or we might put one third of our concentration into each of our Three Tan T'ien. In Chi Kung we can decide what level of attention to direct to any given area of our lives, and how long to maintain it there.

Volume Control is the ability to change the quantity, amount, and intensity of something. In Chi Kung terms this means that you can do a practice lightly or strongly, with full force or with hardly any. You can turn it down or turn it up, as with the volume on a sound system, to get it at just the right volume for any given situation. We have control over just how much of our energy we need or want to use.

ENERGY

AND LIFE

16 Chi Kung and its Applications

A COMPLETE TOOLBOX

Chi Kung can be used for many purposes and all kinds of reasons. It is like a toolbox in which there are many different tools, all with different applications. Some of them are simple and straightforward, while others are so complicated that you need specialized instruction from someone who is trained and experienced. It is as important to pick the right tool as it is to understand the method of using it—you would be as ill-advised to attempt to loosen a screw with a spanner as you would to enter a martial arts competition having only trained in a Chi Kung method for longevity.

By and large, the more simple and broad-based something is, then the more people who are able to do it; the more refined and specialized the thing is, then the fewer people who are interested in it or who can gain access to it. Millions of people can do simple standing postures and they will require minimal instruction, while only the very select few are initiated into the higher levels of Inner Alchemy in the monastic tradition of spiritual cultivation.

Information available nowadays ranges from widely available books; video tapes demonstrating each move of a particular Chi Kung form; weekly, weekend or extended courses, workshops, and training programs. There are programs of every shape and size offered by teachers of various levels of experience and accomplishment (*see* pages 197–198).

A COMPENDIUM OF APPLICATIONS

The following is a compendium of the applications of Chi Kung. Some of them may seem so obvious or mundane that you may question why they are included; others may seem quite fantastic, leading you to wonder how they can be possible.

- Fitness and Sports;
- Martial Arts;
- Health and Healing;
- Sex;
- Longevity;
- Extraordinary Human Abilities;
- Spiritual Development;
- Immortality.

Chi Kung for Fitness and Sports

There are many applications of Chi Kung for fitness. Saying that you are using Chi for fitness in China is like saying you use muscles for exercise in the West—it is nonsensical to try to separate the two. Long established in the East at all levels of society—from morning "stretches" to full workouts—this form of exercise is swiftly entering the mainstream in the West. In YMCAs and health clubs, there is information about alternative exercises, right there among the hi-tech equipment. This information not only covers the three widely familiar disciplines—Yoga, Karate, and Tai Chi—but now also Chi Kung.

There are classic sets for health and fitness—self-massage, The Eight Pieces of Brocade (Ba Duan Jin), The Five Animal Frolics (Wu Qin Xi), Wild Goose Chi Kung, Flying Crane Chi Kung, Swimming Dragon Chi Kung—specific exercise sequences each with its own purpose and benefits.

Chi Kung and the Martial Arts

The martial arts are peculiar to the East. Although all other cultures have fighting forms, in China they have been elevated to a national obsession. There seems to be little history of competitive sports in China. The development of excellence in physical culture is concentrated into fighting, to the extent that it is considered an art form. These days nobody gets hurt very much, but it was not always the way.

Following the arrival of Ta Mo from India, around AD500, at the Shaolin monastery, the monks began to cultivate physical strength through the Muscle Change and Bone Marrow Washing practice (which uses methods to clean accumulated fat from the center of the bones and thereby produce plentiful clean, fresh blood cells—one of the "secrets" of longevity.) They also developed Iron Shirt training, in order to be able to withstand hard blows without damaging essential internal organs. The Shaolin monastery became famous for its martial arts styles, using many secret techniques.

One application of martial arts Chi Kung became known as Hard Chi Kung. Practitioners demonstrate remarkable feats of strength and ability, which are sometimes performed in China as street sideshows for donations from passers-by. Another application is in Tai Chi Chuan, the flowing "shadow boxing," which was used for combat and fighting.

Chi Kung for Health and Healing

Of the many applications of Chi Kung, this may eventually become the most widely known in the West. In terms of effectiveness, there is little to equal it.

There are a number of forms and styles. "Medical Qigong" (*see* page 142) and "Chi Kung Healing" (*see* page 136) are performed by a practitioner who transmits their energy to a patient. These styles depend on a comprehensive working clinical knowledge of the meridian and energy system, as well as the principles involved in Oriental diagnosis and treatment. "Exercise prescriptions" are given for particular illnesses and diseases. Chinese Chi Kung medical books are full of these exercises and practices.

HEALTH =

Balance,
Free Flow,
Right Quality,
Good Volume, &
Correct Relationships

of the Energy System

Chi Kung is a term that can be used to cover many different forms of therapy. Acupuncture, which also works with body-energy, is the most widespread clinical Chi Kung technique in the West. Because of this close affiliation it may be that acupuncturists will increasingly add the title "Chi Kung Healer" to their business cards, as training becomes more widely available. The closest related disciplines at the present are Healing Touch and Therapeutic Touch (*see* page 76).

Chi Kung and Sex

Sex is one of the most compelling and perplexing aspects of life. It generates excitement, confusion, passion, depression, love, compulsion, and joy. In the Oriental system, one's sexual energy is associated with the primary motivating energy, the biological, animal level of being. This is known as Jing, which is one of the Three Treasures—Jing, Chi, and Shen (*see* page 65.) The retention and cultivation of Jing is seen as essential in order to progress to higher levels of energy and spirit.

Trying to understand sex without including the energy system is like visiting a foreign country without speaking the language—and without a map—but Chi Kung can open up this new world of sexuality. There are two aspects to developing sexuality—"single cultivation" and "dual cultivation" (*see* page 129). As implied, sole cultivation is practiced on one's own; dual cultivation with a partner. The development from the primary biological level, through the emotional level to the cultivation of the spirit can not only end unnecessary confusion and pain, but also bring the greatest possible gift into fruition—our higher Love.

Chi Kung for Longevity

One of the most common stereotypes held of China is that of the "wise old sage." In my experience, it really is difficult to know to the nearest decade how old some Chinese people are. Longevity is one of the great prizes in China, and it demonstrates that you have understood the Tao and lived it. In China, it is said that if you died at 120 then you died young. It is not necessary to become ill just because you have grown old. Instead, it depends on the quality, volume, and purity of your essence, energy, and spirit—your Jing, Chi, and Shen.

Chi Kung and Extraordinary Human Abilities

It is established that certain people have highly developed psychic and paranormal abilities. There are people who can do things for which there are no obvious explanations within the currently accepted laws of physics and science.

In attempting to understand the mechanisms involved with extraordinary abilities, one needs to understand that they are operating at higher levels than normal in terms of our sensory perceptions and experience. While there are only a limited number of sensations and experiences we can normally perceive with our sense organs, extraordinary human abilities are related to the ability to perceive at broader, higher, and finer levels.

Through practice and cultivation it is possible to "tune" our sensory apparatus to different frequencies. Using advanced Chi Kung it is possible to perform marvelous activities, such as creating a field of energy which can fill auditoriums and sports stadiums. We all have the inherent potential to develop these abilities.

Chi Kung and Spiritual Development

Spiritual cultivation is part of all cultures, and each society has individual ways and means of approaching it. Many cultures protect their spiritual secrets, and often these are esoteric and only revealed to the initiated. Within Chi Kung these esoteric practices are known as "Inner Alchemy" (*see* page 20), and they are practices that develop heightened states of being. Many means have been used to protect this knowledge, and it is only relatively recently that ancient texts have become available in the West, and that Eastern teachers have been prepared to pass on their knowledge to selected Western students.

In the Taoist tradition, there are considered to be three bodies—the physical body, the soul body, and the spirit body. Each one can be cultivated through specific practices. In order to cultivate the spirit body, Taoist monks refine and purify their physical bodies, thereby raising their energy-bodies to a higher frequency and volume.

Chi Kung and Immortality

The pursuit of Immortality is a central theme of Chi Kung. It is rooted in the most ancient traditions of China and goes back to the earliest shamanic tradition. These traditions include descriptions of the Hsien, the immortals who lived on sunlight, and traveled to the edges of the universe at will.

The actual procedure, which is kept a close secret, involves condensing the energy-body into a "pearl." This pearl is the condensed essence of what we are, the purified stuff of the universe that we each have inside us, the spark of starlight that we call "life." The spirit or essence can then be trained to leave or re-enter the body, through the Chi Kung point called Paihui, at the top of the crown, while the physical body remains in deep meditation.

When it is time to finally leave forever, the practitioner has complete control over the process, and can choose the exact time at which to depart. The pearl/spirit then leaves the body for good, and the physical body "dies."

Inner Alchemy and Spiritual Development

The Master Who Embraces Simplicity, Ge Hong, the most ancient and revered master of longevity and immortality.

It is a beautiful morning in the spring of the 3038th year since the ascension of the Yellow Emperor, the year of the Dragon. On a mist-enshrouded mountain in eastern China, shaped like the spine of a sleeping dragon, Master Ge Hong is climbing the path to his favorite spot for the morning practice of gathering and cultivating universal life force, the Chi. Within his own lifetime he is a famous immortal. He is a master of the Taoist arts of longevity, medicine, and spiritual alchemy.

He has just ingested his strong morning tea of ginseng, tang kuei, three fungi (reishi, ganoderma, and fuling), litchi berries, deer antler, and ho shao wu. Today he will practice a form of self-cultivation called "absorbing celestial nourishment" which is a combination of gentle movements requiring balance and flexibility, visualizations, and the regulation of the breath. He will then stand quietly in deep meditation and merge with invisible forces and realms through ecstatic, transcendent flight. In the 21st century of the Roman calendar (nearly 2,000 years later) these practices will be known throughout the world as Chi Kung.

Master Ge is not simply a man standing in the dawn. He is a local expression of the entire universe. He is the presence within a discrete being of what Taoist writers call "undifferentiated origin" or the "supreme ultimate." He is immortal because he is aware of his unity with what physicists have found to be the timeless and boundless field of infinite possibilities.

OUTER ALCHEMY VS. INNER ALCHEMY

Whether the goal is healthy longevity or immortality, for centuries there has been a debate in China as to whether the supreme elixir is best produced in an external laboratory or in a metaphorical internal laboratory. Ge Hong was an expert in both. The Nei Dan, internal elixir, tradition goes deep into the era of shamanism, long before written history. The Wei Dan, external elixir, tradition began a few generations before Ge Hong was born and it continued through the Tang dynasty (AD618–907). Six Tang dynasty emperors died seeking immortality through external alchemy elixirs that contained mercury and other poisonous metallic elements. By the time of the Southern Song dynasty (AD1126), the era of externally produced elixirs had come to a close and the Nei Dan tradition began to experience a magnificent revival.

EXTERNAL ELIXIRS—EXTERNAL ALCHEMY (WEI DAN)

There is a gradient of external elixirs that ranges from a diet of nutritious vegetables and grain, up through medicaments and formulas containing "super foods," such as ginseng and ho shao wu, to the alchemical level where substances such as cinnabar, mercury, and gold were used. The materials needed to prepare a high-grade elixir were very costly, and the cost to employ a master alchemist was high as well. Inner Alchemy does not have this limitation. The elixir of immortality that is produced within the human body is free to everyone.

INTERNAL ELIXIRS—INNER ALCHEMY (NEI DAN)

By the Song period, the elixir was exclusively produced through Inner Alchemy. One legend about why Hangzhou was chosen for the Song capital suggests that the new emperor wanted to be near Master Ge's hermitage. Higher-level practice—chanting, visualization, prayer, and meditation—produce an aspect of the internal elixir that is more transcendental, yet without being toxic or dangerous. In higher Nei Dan cultivation one merges with the field of virtue and beneficence to become as one with the pure field of energy. Practical methods are combined with transcendental methods of cultivating the consciousness that work to create non-local events, miracles, ecstatic flight, and soul purification. This is a virtual state, wherein one is present in the entire universe while simultaneously being present in one local body.

At the present time, Nei Dan continues to evolve, particularly with the spread of Chi Kung throughout the West. Although it is clear that no one has succeeded in gaining physical immortality on the earthly plane, new scientific evidence suggests that inner enhancement does occur through intentful personal practice. There is also a growing hope that certain nutritional supplements (neutraceuticals) will help to extend life and postpone ageing. As the modern world looks for health, healing, longevity, and even immortality, the ancient practices of Master Ge Hong remain powerful resources in this modern era.

Drawing the light of Sun, Moon, and Big Dipper into the Hall of Enlightenment, they enter trances to refine their bodies. Gathering their life-giving exudate from the golden beams of Paradise, they slow down the race toward old age and retain their youth.

Immortality

In the West, the word "immortal" has the single meaning of living forever in one's current physical human form. In China and other ancient cultures, immortality is much more rich and complex—and more possible. In a practical sense, immortality is the conscious awareness of one's universal nature. In the Chinese context, there are five very different notions of being Immortal. These are:

- Virtue Immortal;
- Legend Immortal;
- Eternally Human Immortal;
- Transcendent Immortal;
- Celestial Immortal.

VIRTUE IMMORTAL

A Virtue Immortal is a revered and virtuous person who is usually quite healthy and insightful. Citizens in a neighborhood or region consider such a person to be an "immortal." One fulfills the qualities of a Virtue Immortal by being a model citizen of great "virtue," by fostering beneficence and virtue in the community, and by making simple wisdom available. Even now, in certain neighborhoods in China, you can ask, "Is there an immortal nearby?" and be directed to his or her humble dwelling. On arrival you will find a kind elder who does not seem to worry much about the details of life. Everyone has access to this level of immortality, but there is no practical evidence that being a Virtue Immortal has any particular eternal value.

LEGEND IMMORTAL

A Legend Immortal is one of the traditional immortals of the Taoist philosophical tradition, the "Eight Immortals" (*see* page 11). It is supposed that these eight characters—often depicted in paintings, sculpture, and poetry as traveling together in an open boat on a sea of cosmic possibilities—are actual human beings who lived exemplary lives and graduated to Celestial Immortal status long ago (*see* page 24). In this respect, they are similar to patron saints in the Western tradition. They are archetypal figures representing some of the great human qualities, and are legendary heroes and a heroine of righteous action and beneficence.

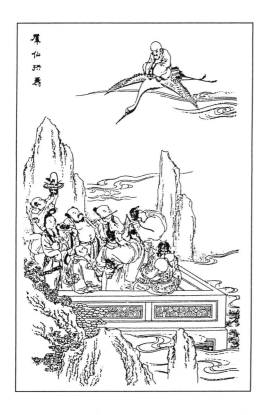

Lao Tzu Flying a Crane to Visit the Eight Immortals

ETERNALLY HUMAN IMMORTAL

An Eternally Human Immortal is one who retains health and youth forever in their human form—physical immortality. This variety of immortality was so alluring to several emperors of China that much of their lifetimes were spent trying to discover the elixir of immortality. Several of them died prematurely from highly toxic formulas containing lethal ingredients. Due to this, the quest for physical immortality fell out of fashion after the Tang dynasty. The idea of living forever in the same physical form is not particularly attractive to most people.

TRANSCENDENT IMMORTAL

A Transcendent Immortal is an individual who has "realized," in their current lifetime, that he or she is a local embodied manifestation of a universal or cosmic resource. This individual is beneficent and spontaneously virtuous because of the profound awareness of the self being fully unified with the entire cosmos, fully woven into the fabric of the One, singular, unitary, cosmic being. Living, realized masters, and profoundly enlightened teachers who are aware of the undifferentiated nature of consciousness, are Transcendent Immortals. In the Buddhist tradition, when such a person dies, the soul may elect to return for additional earthly reincarnations as a Bodhisattva, a compassionate soul who commits to revisit Earthly life until all beings have found peace and ascended into the heavenly realm.

CELESTIAL IMMORTAL

A Celestial Immortal is one who has lived an exemplary life of right action, usually through their understanding of cosmic unity. They have met the Celestial criteria and, at death, will ascend into Heaven to reside as an immortal. The Celestial Immortal is considered a transcendent expression of the personal self—so personal characteristics are retained in the celestial realm. Transcendent Immortals, following the completion of their local lives, typically become Celestial Immortals. The Taoist Celestial Immortal ascends into a layered multitude of heavens, as did both the Yellow Emperor and Ge Hong.

THE QUEST FOR IMMORTALITY

In a modern, scientific sense, it can be said that it is impossible *not* to be immortal. Quantum science suggests that time and space are illusions based on the limitations of human sensory and intellectual capacity, and that in reality we dwell in a boundless and timeless quantum field. Most religions promise some sort of eternal life, through a combination of right action and devotional practice—"The spirit never dies and the soul is eternal." Whether one is admitted to Heaven by grace or by working through karma and reincarnation, everlasting life is generally guaranteed.

Chi Kung Today and Scientific Research

Chi Kung is entering into the West at an incredible speed. Thanks to computers and digital technology, long-held secrets are now instantaneously available and disseminated. In these stressful times, there is more need than ever for inward focus, peace, and inner knowledge.

The first books explaining in plain language some of the primary practices appeared in English in the mid 1980s. There are now hundreds of books on every possible aspect of Chi Kung practice from basic introductions to the most advanced practice. More and more people are specializing in Chi Kung Healing or adding it to their existing practices in acupuncture, massage, bodywork, and other disciplines. There are personal instructors who offer individual training, and residential retreat centers that specialize in nothing else.

National and International Associations are blossoming forth like flowers. In the United States, the National Qigong (Chi Kung) Association ∗ USA was formed in 1996; it now has members throughout the USA. In Europe, the European Federation of Tai Chi and Qigong has 18 member countries and the European Federation of Medical Qigong includes medical doctors as members. In China, the World Academic Society of Medical Qigong represents 24 countries, all of which have agreed to a basic curriculum of training, and it holds international conferences where the majority of the attendees are doctors or research scientists. There is discussion, exchange visits, information, and dialogue taking place on a global scale.

On a local level, not very long ago Chi Kung practices may have seemed strange, but they are now appearing on the programs of health clubs everywhere. Psychologists are beginning to integrate "energy work" into their practices—Chi Kung and Tai Chi have been taught in high-security prisons, with a consequent reduction of inmate violence—and the orthodox medical world is paying careful attention because of the undeniable clinical results. Chi Kung is coming of age and it feels as though we are in the midst of a "Chi Revolution." But is there any concrete proof of its efficacy?

MEDICAL SCIENCE AND RESEARCH

One of the more exciting advances in healthcare today is the integration of Western and Chinese medicine. As cultures share information, medicine can evolve to provide more effective healthcare. For instance, clinical studies have shown that patients who practice Chi Kung can reverse symptoms of ageing, have fewer strokes, and live longer. In the early 1980s, scientists in China began to study the medical benefits claimed for Chi Kung and, since then, research on hundreds of medical applications of Chi Kung have been reported. Details of this research can be found in the Computerized Qigong Database created by Dr. Kenneth Sancier of The Qigong Institute in California (see details on page 188).

Many of the studies are designed to show the effects of emitted Chi on living systems, and on the functions and organs of the human body. Some of these, and the measurement techniques employed (in parenthesis), include:

- **Brain (EEG and magnetometer);**
- **Blood flow (thermography, sphygmography, and rheoencephalography);**
- **Heart functions (blood pressure, EKG, and UCG);**
- **Kidney (urinary albumin assay);**
- **Biophysical (enzyme activity, immune function, sex hormone levels);**
- **Eyesight (clinical);**
- **Tumor size in mice.**

26   Several clinical studies have specifically addressed the benefits of Chi Kung for alleviating or reversing the symptoms of ageing. Research has been carried out at the Shanghai Institute of Hypertension that can be seen as a model for ways in which Chi Kung can improve the functions and organs of the body. Hypertension (high blood pressure) is one major medical problem in the West, causing deterioration of vital organs and their functions, leading to premature ageing. In the Shanghai study it was demonstrated that Chi Kung can significantly help reduce blood pressure, mortality, and stroke; improve heart function and micro-circulation; improve sex hormone levels and blood chemistry.

The main conclusion from many scientific and medical research studies is that Chi Kung exercise can help the body heal itself. Chi Kung is a natural anti-ageing medicine, and there are many medical applications of Chi Kung that can complement Western medicine to improve healthcare.

PART TWO

Your Energy System

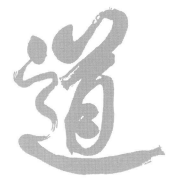

CHAPTER THREE

Chi and the Energy System

氣功

Understanding Chi

WHAT IS IN A NAME?

Some Chinese words, such as Yin, Yang, and Tai Chi, simply cannot be translated into other languages; they stand in their own right. When words are translated from one language into the primary language of another culture, then often the best approximate word meaning the same thing is used. "Chair" is easily translated because it is a solid object that most people use. Unlike chairs, though, some words are not part of our culture, and so are less easy to translate. "Chi" is one such word.

The closest approximation to Chi in the English language is "energy." This is the translation that has entered into common usage, but what does "energy" mean in this context? It has been described by other words, such as "vitality," "élan vital," and "prana" but these are rather awkward, self-conscious, or simply miss the point.

One difficulty is that most people have never consciously experienced and differentiated Chi, because they have never practiced or studied Chi Kung. If you have not experienced something, it is a struggle to understand the concept. If you asked a fish in a bowl what the water was like, the fish would have no idea what you were talking about, because it would have no idea of what it means not to be in water.

It is similar with Chi. It is everywhere, in everything, within us and all around us. It is all-pervasive, omnipresent, and ineffable. Descriptions of this quality are similar to qualities ascribed to God or the Divine. So, part of our problem with the word "Chi" is that it is beyond our language, and another is that it is beyond our experience.

Another word that can be used to describe what we mean by "energy," is "life." While it is understandable, it may be one of our greatest oversights and losses to miss this point, that it is possible that "energy" and "life" are effectively the same thing. It is like saying "food," but not knowing anything about farming, gardening, cooking, or seasoning; saying "dance," but not knowing any of the steps or rhythms. It is similar to performing a simple act, such as walking, without knowing anything of the muscles, nerves, or bones and their inter-relationships.

EXPERIENCING CHI

So what is this Chi or energy that is everywhere and within everything? How do we experience it, and how does it manifest itself? The experience of Chi has most often been described as a flowing current.

This may be because of our experience of flowing water, how we feel the flow of water over our skin. If you pour some warm water on the top of your arm, you feel it flow down the arm to the hand and fingertips. When you swim or bathe in warm water, it produces a particular sensation on the surface of the body. A flowing current is similar—it is a sensation of something moving from one place to another. It has a distinct feeling and is a specific event. It is like "mains hum," the basic energetic level of what is in us—the "buzz" of life itself.

The effect of Chi during Acupuncture treatment can be felt by quadriplegics—people who have suffered severe injury to the central nervous system—even though they experience no feeling in the body or limbs deriving from the action of the nerves.

BETTER ENERGY—BETTER LIFE

Chi can also have particular qualities—it can feel heavy or light, full or empty, thick or thin, and so on. If you pay attention you will find words to describe your experience. To increase your energy is like increasing the brightness and luminosity—as if turning up a dimmer switch from low to bright.

People with the best body-energy, function on a higher frequency energy field. Not only do they have more energy, function at a higher level, and stay healthier, but also people of lower energy level are attracted to them. This may be the mysterious "charisma" often attributed to those such as leaders, stars of theatre or screen, healers, and spiritual teachers.

The stronger and better the quality of our energy, the more successful we are in life. This also applies to optimism, being full of spirit and positive feelings, brimming with life, and it is the opposite of depression, hopelessness, and lifelessness. Energy is the antidote of everything that we do not want.

People with illnesses have low energy fields and "bad" energy. In a culture that does not have an understanding of this, it is no wonder that many of the commonly occurring mental, emotional, and psychological ills are treated with chemicals, pharmaceuticals, and psychotherapy—too often with no noticeable success. Indeed, these approaches can often make things a great deal worse.

If there is an energy problem, then it requires an energy solution. Nothing else will do the trick. So we need to identify the correct and specific energy issue, and adjust it accordingly. This is not to disregard the enormous importance of biological and medical science, but to incorporate the reality of the energy system into the picture. Without doing this we are playing with half of a deck, because we are not including an essential reality that underlies and pervades everything.

Chi Kung is a way to activate, cleanse, purify, refine, increase, heighten, circulate, and store our energy. It is a way to keep it in correct balance, flow, quality, volume, and relationships and it is under our conscious control.

People engage in many activities in order to optimize their energetic state. These usually involve some kind of physical or meditative activity, and the desired effect is often a by-product or purely accidental. Instead, it makes sense to go directly to the core experience itself by practicing a specific, time-limited activity that corrects your energy and state of being. This also applies if it is for a specific purpose—to correct or dispel a physical symptom, or an emotional or mental state.

Whatever the motive, through practicing Chi Kung you are likely to have a new experience of yourself—in the same way you feel refreshed after a shower, stimulated after swimming in warm clear water, or exhilarated when standing on a hilltop after a pleasant climb. You will have experiences of your own which relate to what it feels like when you are at your best.

The Anatomy and Physiology of the Energy System

In the human body, Chi has an anatomy and physiology that follow a set of rules and laws that are as strict and fixed as those in Western anatomy and physiology. Chi is the foundation of Acupuncture, it is what medicinal herbs act upon, and it is what practices such as Chi Kung affect and develop.

The Oriental view of anatomy and physiology is that our state of health is based in our meridian system, and that our Chi can be guided and developed—internally by the mind and externally by movement. It is essential for anyone wishing to understand Chi Kung to have a basic guide map of the anatomy (structure) and physiology (function) of the energy system. Many of the concepts are unfamiliar to the Western way of thinking, and there are numerous words and names for the same thing, which differ according to the particular source or translation. However, a broad sketch of the landscape will help us to find our way around.

ENERGY ANATOMY

Knowledge of the energy anatomy provides a foundation for an understanding that has been the basis of healthcare and general well-being for millions of Chinese and Asian people throughout recorded history. The main features of this energy anatomy system are:

- The Meridians;
- The Organs and the Officials;
- The Points;
- The Three Chou;
- The Pulses;
- The Basic Substances (Chi, Blood, and Fluids);
- The Three T'ien;
- The Three Treasures;
- Soul and Spirit.

The Meridians

The meridians are channels or pathways in the body along which the Chi flows. The meridians are a separate and discrete system, independent of any of the other anatomical systems. In total there are 35 meridians and together they constitute the complete anatomy of the Chi meridian system. This comprises:

- Twelve major meridians;
- Eight Extraordinary meridians;
- Fifteen collateral channels.

The twelve major meridians, plus the two main Extraordinary meridians, constitute the 14 major channels, and along them they have a differing number of "energy points." These are the points where acupuncture, heat, massage, or some other form of stimulation is applied to effect changes in the energy system. Together they connect every part of the body as an integrated whole. The Chi flows out from these major channels to the rest of the body—to our cells, tissues, and organs.

The Organs and the Officials

The 12 main meridians are each related to a particular organ. Traditionally, these organs are not considered just to be the physical organ, but rather each one is seen as an "official." Each official has responsibility for, and control over, a particular domain or function, just as in society people have certain areas of responsibility.

The Points

The other aspect of the anatomy of the energy system that is critical to understanding how the energy operates is the "points." These are specific places on the surface of the body where the energy can be affected and changed, most familiar and well-known through acupuncture. There are 670 commonly agreed points along the meridians, together with the Extraordinary and "New" points.

The Chi Kung points

In Chi Kung there are certain major points that are used regularly by all practitioners (see diagram on page 34). They are:

- The navel;
- The rear navel;
- The crown;
- The perineum;
- The palms;
- The soles of the feet;
- The heart point;
- The rear heart;
- The brow;
- The tip of the tongue.

It is necessary to have a working knowledge and understanding of these major points in order to progress beyond repetitive learning. This is covered in more detail later (see page 60).

The Three Chou

Another important and unique structure of Oriental anatomy is the way in which the torso is divided into three separate sections. These are known as The Three Chou. The lower Chou is the area below the navel. The middle Chou is from the navel to the diaphragm at the base of the rib cage. The upper Chou is the area from the diaphragm to the neck. Each of these areas

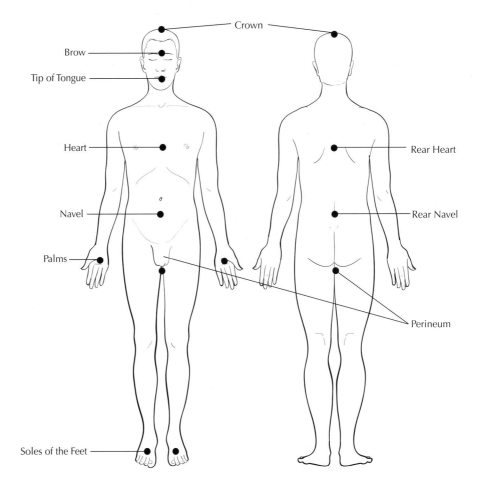

The 12 Primary Chi Kung Points

operates at a separate and independent temperature, and each governs the particular internal organs and functions in that area, so the correct balance and integration between them is essential.

The Pulses

The pulses are the basic way in which the Chi in the 12 major meridians, and therefore a person's energy, is read and monitored. Each of the 12 organs/officials has a separate and distinct pulse, which can be felt and "read" by the fingertips of a trained and experienced practitioner. These pulses are located on the radial artery of the wrist, and they may also be felt at the ankle and neck.

There are three positions on each wrist, the first at the normal position for feeling the heart-rate pulse, opposite the styloid process, the second postion is one fingertip in front of this, and the third position one fingertip behind. In each position there are two levels—one superficial, the other deep, so there are six positions on each wrist, making a total of 35 12 pulses altogether.

Each of these pulses is classically described as having 27 different qualities that can be felt, and these are described in terms such as floating or sinking, hard or soft, fast or slow, large or small, full or empty. There are also combinations of these qualities. In this way it is possible to know the nature of the Chi in a particular organ, and therefore its state and condition. This is a most revealing and comprehensive technique, and it is limited only by the skill and experience of the practitioner.

The Basic Substances—Chi, Blood and Fluids

Chi, Blood, and Fluids are the fundamental substances in the human body. They are derived from the essence of breathing, eating, and drinking—the usual ways in which we take in energy from the outside (external Chi)—and they sustain normal vital functions, nourishing and lubricating the organs and tissues. The quality of the Chi determines the quality of the blood and fluids, and the quality of the blood and fluids determines the quality of the Chi; stagnation in one will cause stagnation in the other. Both are food for our cells, so having good quality in them is essential for health and vitality.

The Three Tan T'ien

The Three Tan T'ien are also known as the Three Fields of Cultivation. This refers to three areas of the body—on the lower abdomen where one's power is stored (the lower Tan T'ien), on the middle abdomen where one's emotions and Chi reside (the middle Tan T'ien), and in the center of the head where mental and spiritual dimensions are developed (the upper Tan T'ien). These are the areas where The Three Treasures are cultivated.

The Three Treasures

At a more basic level, underlying all of these structures and functions is the way in which the Chinese understand the totality of the human being. They categorize us as having three basic components known as The Three Treasures, and a depletion or deficiency in any of these will undermine the whole of our being. These are called:

- Jing;
- Chi;
- Shen.

Soul and Spirit

Spirit and Soul are terms used in the West for which there is no commonly accepted overall definition. In the Oriental tradition there are various subtle distinctions to what we call the Spirit and Soul in the West. There are understood to be five aspects of the Spirit and Soul and each one is related to an organ/official, as shown in the table on page 36.

CHI AND THE

ENERGY SYSTEM

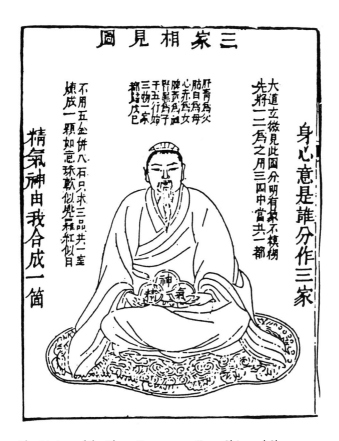

The Union of the Three Treasures—Jing, Chi, and Shen

SPIRIT/SOUL	ORGAN/OFFICIAL
Hun	Liver
Shen	Heart
Yi	Spleen
Po	Lungs
Zhi	Kidneys

By purifying, nourishing, and refining these organs/officials through specific formulas and procedures, one develops the Virtues, each of which is an expression of the Spirit and Soul. This is the foundation for the spiritual tradition and practice of Chi Kung.

The physiology of the energy system is a reflection of its laws and principles. These are based on the laws of nature and Chi Kung operates according to these laws. The major features are:

- The Tao;
- Yin and Yang (and the Eight Principles);
- The Five Elements;
- Family Relationships;
- The Table of Correspondence;
- The Factors of Disease;
- Natural Cycles and Biorhythms—the Earth, Moon, and Sun.

Understanding and recognizing each of these gives us a deep sense of our inherent functioning and how we are intrinsically connected to the whole of nature, and it also indicates what we may do to align ourselves with it.

The Tao

Our physiology operates according to the principles of The Tao (The Way) (*see* page 9). This is the origin and the nature of all things. Chi Kung could be described as "The Tao in Action."

Yin and Yang, and the Eight Principles

The symbol of The Tao is seen in the familiar image of the two interlocking fishes. One is white and the other is black and they represent the basic polarity of opposites, known as the Yin and the Yang. This polarity encompasses everything.

To our common perception, everything is complemented by its opposite—up/down, black/white, day/night, positive/negative, male/female, movement/stillness, and growth/decay. These principles all operate according to specific natural laws. The most fundamental of these are the laws of Yin and Yang.

Yin and Yang polarity forms the basis of what is known as the Eight Principles. This is a way of understanding and describing the state and condition of the Chi according to eight parameters. These form four pairs of opposites:

- Yin = Yang;
- Interior = Exterior;
- Deficient = Excessive;
- Cold = Hot.

For instance, a person may have an internal energy condition that could be described as "yin, interior, deficient, and cold" or "yang, exterior, excessive, and hot." In a practical sense, this allows for a way of thinking about a specific condition, which enables a practitioner to be able to decide on a course of action that would resolve the differences and bring the opposites back into balance.

Five major principles of Yin/Yang have been recognized, which describe their interaction:

1   Everything has a Yin and Yang aspect;
2   Every Yin and Yang can be further divided;
3   Yin and Yang create each other;
4   Yin and Yang control each other;
5   Yin and Yang can each transform into the other.

The Five Elements—Wood, Fire, Earth, Metal, and Water

After the division into Yin and Yang, the Taoists divide all things into the Five Elements. This is a way of understanding and describing the nature of things in categories according to their inherent qualities. There are many ways in which the Five Elements interact together, and these differences form the basis for whole schools of thought in Taoism.

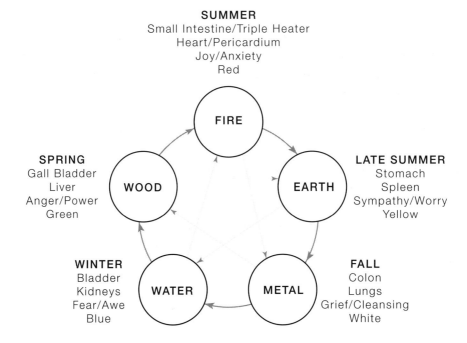

SUMMER
Small Intestine/Triple Heater
Heart/Pericardium
Joy/Anxiety
Red

SPRING
Gall Bladder
Liver
Anger/Power
Green

LATE SUMMER
Stomach
Spleen
Sympathy/Worry
Yellow

WINTER
Bladder
Kidneys
Fear/Awe
Blue

FALL
Colon
Lungs
Grief/Cleansing
White

FIRE
WOOD
EARTH
WATER
METAL

The Five Elements and their Main Correspondences—Seasons, Organs, Emotions, and Colors

It is perhaps easiest to understand the Five Elements in relationship to the seasons of the year. The succession of the seasons is the basic condition under which all life evolves. This is so fundamental that we tend not to notice it. The seasons are based on the rotation of the Earth around the Sun. They always follow the same sequence, and never miss a season or go in the opposite direction. They are stable and predictable, and provide the metronome of life. Although in the West we consider there to be four seasons, particularly in temperate climates, the Orientals have five. While the familiar Western sequence is Spring, Summer, Fall, and Winter, the Orientals consider the period of Late Summer (sometimes called Indian Summer) to be a distinct season of its own. It is the point of balance and harmony of the year—the Center Place.

Each of the seasons has a particular quality that reflects its character and nature. Each of these qualities is described in terms of an Element or Phase—Wood, Fire, Earth, Metal, and Water.

- **Wood is the power or force which motivates things to grow in the Spring;**
- **Fire is the heat and activity which reaches a peak in Summer;**
- **Earth is the ground which provides a foundation for everything, reaching the center point of Late Summer;**
- **Metal is the minerals which return to the ground in Fall;**
- **Water is the snow and ice of Winter.**

The Five Elements and seasons also have corresponding organs and emotions (*see* page 41). In addition to all of this there are many more relationships of the Five Elements, given in The Table of Correspondences on page 40. These relationships are expanded into many other aspects of life, and they provide the basic foundation for this comprehensive and integrated way of experiencing the world.

The Table of Correspondences is the classical Oriental way of understanding our holistic nature and the relationship between all our parts. This way of seeing things ties all of the different aspects of ourselves into an integrated whole. For example, the physical level of organs, senses, tissues, functions; the emotional level of our basic feelings; the mental level of our abilities of planning, decision making, willpower, differentiation, and control; and the various dimensions and levels of the human spirit. The Table also extends into the relationships of such things as colors, sounds, odors, times of day, and flavors. It is an understanding of the relationships of all our parts, and is one of the original holistic views of the world.

ELEMENT	WOOD	FIRE	EARTH	METAL	WATER
SEASON	Spring	Summer	Late summer	Autumn	Winter
YANG ORGAN	Gall Bladder	Small Intestine Three Heater	Stomach	Colon	Bladder
YIN ORGAN	Liver	Heart Pericardium	Spleen	Lungs	Kidneys
EMOTION	Anger/Power	Joy/Anxiety	Sympathy/Worry	Grief/Cleansing	Fear/Awe
COLOR	Green	Red	Yellow	White	Blue
SOUND	Shouting	Laughing	Singing	Weeping	Groaning
TASTE	Sour	Bitter	Sweet	Pungent	Salty
SMELL	Rancid	Scorched	Fragrant	Rotten	Putrid
OPENING	Eyes	Tongue	Mouth	Nose	Ears
TISSUE	Tendons	Blood Vessels	Flesh	Skin and Hair	Bones
CLIMATE	Wind	Heat	Damp	Dry	Cold
PROCESS	Birth	Growth	Transformation	Harvest	Storage
DIRECTION	East	South	Center	West	North

The Table of Correspondences

Family Relationships

A number of the basic laws and principles of the meridian system reflect the relationships of our most fundamental unit—the family. This is based upon the cycle of the Five Elements.

Mother–Child

The Law of Mother–Child is one of the principles of Taoist philosophy that are based on the most obvious relationships and patterns in the ordinary everyday world. It is also known as the Shen or Nurturing Cycle. In its simplest form it states that each organ/official is the mother of the organ/official following it, and the child of the one preceding it. According to the cycle, each official is "fed" or nurtured by the official that precedes it, just as a mother is responsible for nourishing her child. Therefore, if the mother is not functioning in a healthy way—is either too weak or too strong—then the child will be correspondingly affected, and vice versa.

There are also permutations of Grandmother–Grandchild that operate in a similar way.

The Husband–Wife Law

The relationship of husband–wife/man–woman is the foundation from which we all come. To the Taoist viewpoint this is a reflection of the relationship between Yin and Yang, and this has to have a particular dynamic and balance in order for movement to take place. If Yin and

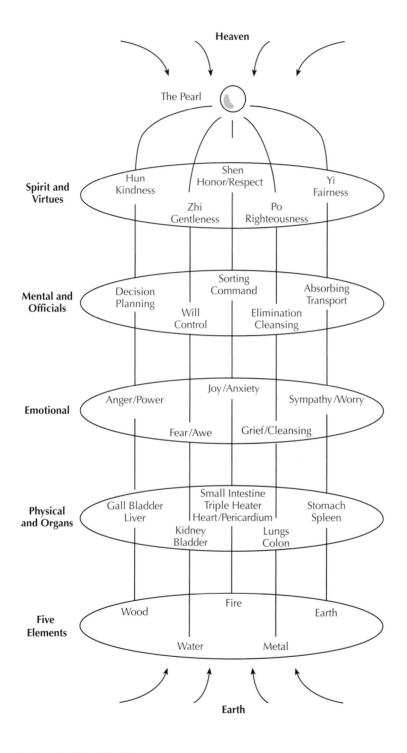

The Five levels of the Five Elements

Yang are perfectly balanced there would be no activity, only stagnation. To be in the correct balance the Yang has to be slightly stronger than the Yin. If the Yin is stronger than the Yang then the dynamic is not correct and this is a serious condition which, if not corrected, may lead to chaos, because the natural, inherent dynamic is reversed. Similarly, according to this principle, in a male–female, husband–wife relationship the man should manifest yang and the woman manifest yin, in order to sustain a harmonious relationship.

Brothers and Sisters

All organs are paired in couples, according to their Five Element relationship. These are Liver and Gall Bladder in Wood, Heart and Small Intestine, Pericardium and Triple Heater in Fire, Spleen and Stomach in Earth, Lungs and Colon in Metal, and Kidneys and Bladder in Water. These couples have a Sister–Brother/Yin–Yang relationship.

The Causes of Disease

So where does imbalance and disease come from, and why does Chi become dysfunctional? There are two basic causes of disease—external and internal.

External factors can include: adverse environmental conditions of heat, cold, damp, wind, dryness, and humidity; wrong diet; spoiled food; worms and microbes; poisoning and pollution; trauma and accidents.

Internal conditions can arise from excess or deficient emotions of anger, joy, sympathy, grief, or fear. These can be generated from the emotional environment you are in, or can be caused by inappropriate mental attitudes and beliefs. There are also maladies of the spirit. All of these factors can cause one's Chi to become excessive, deficient, stuck, blocked, congested, or stagnant, thereby leading to all manner of problems. Knowing and understanding these factors, and then avoiding them, can be a major aspect of preserving your Chi. An overall understanding of the anatomy and physiology of the energy system helps to maintain and develop one's health and state of being.

Natural Cycles and Biorhythms—the Earth, Moon, and Sun

Many aspects of the body are based on natural cycles—the rhythms and regularities of nature. Our bodies evolved over millions of years within the context of the Earth, Moon, and Sun cycles. We experience these from our own perspective as the alternations of day and night, the monthly Moon cycle, and the cycle of the seasons. We are profoundly affected by these rhythms as they come and go, and by understanding these cycles we can attune ourselves to the inherent rhythms of our own energy as it moves inside us, and thereby attune to nature.

The Earth and Day/Night

In the West, there are 24 hours in each day, and there are 12 major organs in the body. Chi flows in the meridians and organs continuously, but it reaches a peak level in each organ for about two hours each day, moving like a tidal wave through all of the organs. This is the same for everyone and the movement is related to the relative position of the Sun. So, at specific times of the day, it is possible to affect the relevant organ more than at others. The time is in relationship to Sun time, and should therefore be adjusted accordingly in countries that move the time one hour forward for "Summer Time." There are particular energy points—one on each meridian—which can be used to activate the organ/official at the that time; these are called the Horary points. In fact, the ancient Chinese clock consisted of just twelve units in a day, with each unit consisting of two of our contemporary hours, as follows:

ORGAN	PEAK TIME	CHINESE NAME
Heart	11am–1pm	Wu
Small Intestine	1pm–3pm	Wei
Bladder	3pm–5pm	Shen
Kidneys	5pm–7pm	You
Pericardium	7pm–9pm	Xu
Triple Heater	9pm–11pm	Hai
Gall Bladder	11pm–1am	Zi
Liver	1am–3am	Chou
Lungs	3am–5am	Yin
Colon	5am–7am	Mao
Stomach	7am–9am	Chen
Spleen	9am–11am	Si

This reflects the biological fact of energy movement in our bodies and organs. The significance and importance of this is considerable as it affects all of our daily functions, abilities, and moods.

The Moon and the Month

Every monthly Moon cycle the Chi completes one circulation up the back and down the front of the body, through the Governor and Conception channels. At the Full moon, the Chi is at its peak, the crown of the head. At the New Moon it is at the perineum. This monthly Moon circulation controls the tides and is the basis of women's menstrual cycles.

The Sun and the Seasons

In each season the Chi also reaches a peak in a pair of organs, as follows:

SPRING	Gall Bladder and Liver
SUMMER	Small Intestine and Heart
LATE SUMMER	Stomach and Spleen
FALL	Colon and Lungs
WINTER	Bladder and Kidneys

In this way the Seasons have a profound effect on us. Most doctors are aware from experience that certain organs have symptoms at particular times of the year, and this circulation of energy is the reason why.

The Eight Diagrams

The Eight Diagrams or "Pa Kua" is a system of understanding that describes the basic nature of change, how it works, and how to work with it. It is a diagram of the primary dynamics of reality.

The Pa Kua consists of eight sets of three lines. The top line represents Heaven. The bottom line represents Earth. The middle line represents Humankind. These are known as the "trigrams." These lines can be either Yang, which are unbroken, or Yin, which are broken.

Yang   Yin

The two primary trigrams are full Yang and full Yin—representing Heaven and Earth. When any of these lines change into their opposite, they create one of six possible permutations—Thunder, Water, Mountain, Wind, Fire, and Lake.

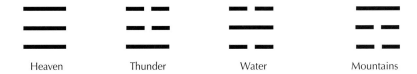

Heaven   Thunder   Water   Mountains

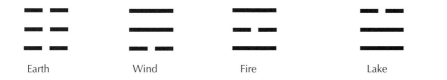

| Earth | Wind | Fire | Lake |

The trigrams can be placed in particular relationships to each other in the form of an eight-sided figure—the Pa Kua. The position and relationship in the octagon reflects particular dynamics between the primary trigrams, so that they describe different versions of the dynamics of reality.

There are two primary arrangements of the Pa Kua—Earlier Heaven (Ho Tu) and Later Heaven (Lo Shu). Ho Tu means Yellow River Plan, and was said to be seen by the legendary Emperor Fu Hi as spots on the back of a dragon-horse rising out of the Ho river. Lo Shu means Lo River Writing and, according to legend, the Emperor Yu is said to have discovered it on the back of a tortoiseshell. These configurations relate to how the energy circulates in the embryo and before birth (pre-natal circulation) and after birth (post-natal circulation). They are the primary descriptions of the circulation of energy.

This is reflected in the Microcosmic Orbit meditation (*see* pages 99), where the Chi is directed from the navel, down the front of the abdomen, to the perineum, then up the center of the back to the crown and over the head to descend down the middle of the front, back to the navel. This is the circulation of the Chi in the womb, when all energy from the mother enters into the child through the umbilical cord at the navel.

At the moment of birth, the umbilical cord is cut and the energy in the child begins to operate on its own. The Chi contracts into the lower abdomen, in the lower Tan T'ien. It then descends internally to the perineum and splits in two directions, with one ascending the Conception channel up the front of the torso to the bottom lip; the other ascends the back, up the Governor channel, and over the top of the head, down to the top lip.

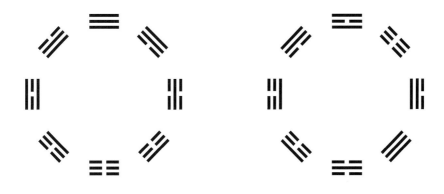

EARLIER HEAVEN PA KUA   **LATER HEAVEN PA KUA**

The child now takes in its external Chi from Heaven and Earth, from breathing and eating, the energy of oxygen and food combining internally to create the Chi that, along with the Yin inherited from the parents and ancestors, runs in the meridians (*see* Jing Chi Shen, page 65).

The practice of the Microcosmic Orbit reverses the post-natal circulation back to the pre-natal circulation, so that instead of dividing at the perineum and running in two directions, up the front and up the back to meet at the mouth, the Chi nows runs from the navel in a complete cycle, down to the perineum, up the back and down the front to finish back at the navel. So, Later Heaven reverts back to Earlier Heaven, thereby restoring the primary energy circulation.

THE I CHING

The trigrams are basic to the *I Ching* (*The Book of Changes*). This is the primary Taoist classic, and the most revered book in Taoist tradition. It has an astounding ability to describe reality on all levels, and it ties together all aspects—personal, emotional, intellectual, spiritual, situational, social, and political—into one integrated, coherent whole.

It has been proposed that the system of logic underlying reality consists of these primary eight patterns and configurations—the eight trigrams. Full Yang and full Yin represent the bookends of reality—it is not possible to go beyond absolute yang or absolute yin. As illustrated above, the other six trigrams (Thunder, Water, Mountain, Wind, Fire, and Lake) represent the possible changes between Yang and Yin.

In the *I Ching* there are eight trigrams depicted on a horizontal axis and eight trigrams on a vertical axis, giving a total of 64 possible combinations of two trigrams—one trigram above and one below—giving a six-line figure (a hexagram). Each hexagram constitutes a separate chapter in the *I Ching*, and it is described and interpreted as to its significance to a person, situation, or circumstance. Using methods such as tossing coins or picking yarrow stalks to select hexagrams, this is also the basis of a powerful ancient divinatory system.

The Pa Kua is a remarkable and mysterious pattern and has many dimensions of interest; but for our purposes, beyond its importance in understanding the Microcosmic Orbit, it is also of great significance in the Eight Extraordinary meridians (*see* page 55).

CHAPTER FOUR

The Meridians and Points

氣功

The meridians and points comprise the primary anatomy of the energy system, the energetic structure through which Chi flows. The network of channels and points that the energy flows through are comparable to the anatomy of blood circulation and the nervous system. They are:

*   The Twelve Major Organ Meridians;
*   The Eight Extraordinary Meridians;
*   The Twelve Primary Chi Kung Points;
*   The Master and Coupled Points;
*   Jing Chi Shen.

The Twelve Major Organ Meridians

There are 12 major energy channels/meridians on the body, each of which relates to a specific organ. They run along the surface of the body in a symmetrical and logical layout.

Along these channels are the "points" which are used in Acupuncture, Chi Kung and Acupressure. Each point has a name and a very specific and, usually, unique function. The points on a given channel affect that particular channel, but they can also have effects on other channels and organs.

Since many forms of Chi Kung automatically have the desired effect on specific points, you do not necessarily need to know the points to get the benefits of the practice. However, it certainly helps to know the pathways, because your mind is involved in moving your Chi. To understand Chi Kung fully, you should know these basic pathways and organs/officials.

In the West, the meridians are usually known by the name of the corresponding organ, but in the classical Chinese view they were seen rather as "officials", in the sense that the body is a self-contained society and each organ had a particular function in relation to the whole.

In the Table of Correspondences, the meridian is not considered to relate solely to that particular organ but to many other aspects of the person as well.

The 12 major organ meridians have both superficial and deep pathways, and there are connecting channels between them. On the superficial level they form a continuous loop or circuit with the end of one flowing into the beginning of the next. Beginning on the torso, the Heart channel flows to the hands where it switches to the Small Intestine channel which then flows from the hands to the head, this switches to the Bladder channel which flows down to the feet, which then switches to the Kidney channel which flows back up to the torso. This circulation of sets of four channels then continues with the Pericardium channel (also known as the Conception/Sex channel), Triple Heater channel (also known as the Three Heater channel), Gall Bladder channel, and Liver channel, then repeats with the Lung channel, Colon channel, Stomach channel, and Spleen channel, ending up on the torso again, and flowing back into the heart channel. These are all bilateral, mirror images of each other on the left and right side.

MERIDIAN NO.	ORGAN	NO. OF POINTS	OFFICIAL
I	Heart	9	Sovereign/Supreme Controller
II	Small Intestines	19	Separating Pure and Impure
III	Bladder	67	Storage of Water
IV	Kidneys	27	Controller of Water
V	Pericardium	9	Heart Protector
VI	Triple Heater	23	Balance and Harmony
VII	Gall Bladder	44	Decisions and Wise Judgment
VIII	Liver	14	Planning/The General
IX	Lungs	11	Receiving Pure Chi from Heaven
X	Colon	20	Great Eliminator/Drainage and Dregs
XI	Stomach	45	Rotting and Ripening
XII	Spleen	21	Transport

These 12 constitute the primary organs/functions. There are also other organs known as the "Peculiar Organs" that are not considered to be discrete and independent since they are affected and influenced by a number of meridians—these include the brain and the uterus.

The Heart Channel

The Heart channel has 9 points. It begins under the armpit, runs down the inside of the inside arm to the elbow, then continues on to the wrist, down the palm to end on the outside nail point of the little finger.

Small Intestine Channel

The Small Intestine channel has 19 points. It begins on the inside nail point of the little finger, proceeds along the edge of the finger, up the inside of the outer arm up to the crease where the arm meets the torso, over the shoulder blade, over the neck to the cheekbone and ends at the ear.

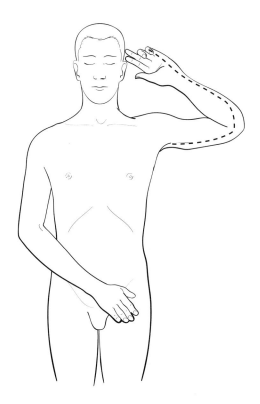

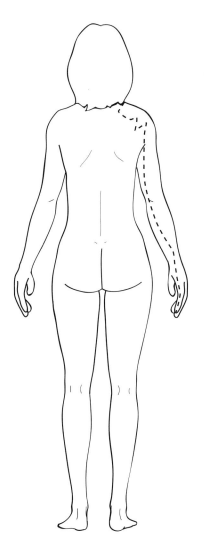

The Bladder Channel

The Bladder channel has 67 points. It begins on the inside corner of the eye, ascends to the top of the eye socket, then over the head to the base of the skull and down the neck to the top of the shoulder. It then splits into two lines which run parallel down the back to the pelvis, join at the buttocks, then continue down the back of the leg to the ankle and along the outside edge of the little toe to end on the outside nail point.

The Kidney Channel

The Kidney channel has 27 points. It begins on the inside nail point of the little toe, moves to the bottom of the foot, ascends over the inside of the foot to the inside ankle, then ascends up the inside leg to the torso and continues in a straight line to end below the collarbone.

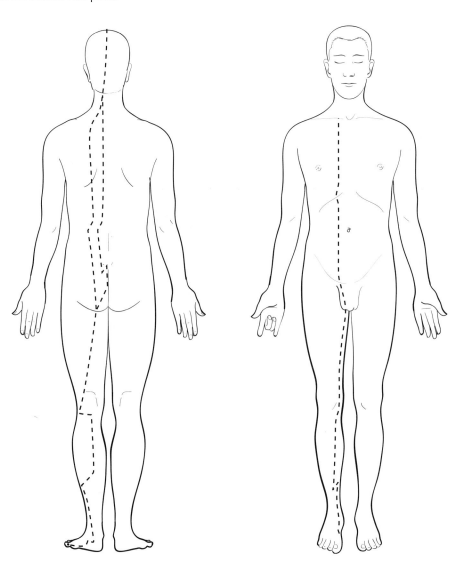

The Pericardium Channel

The Pericardium channel has 9 points. It begins at the outside edge of the nipple, flows up to the top of the arm then runs down the middle of the inside arm, past the elbow and wrist, then down the center of the palm to end on the outside nail point of the second finger.

TheTriple Heater Channel

The Triple Heater (Three Heater) channel has 23 points. It begins on the inside nail point of the fourth finger, ascends up the finger to the middle of the wrist, then up the middle of the outside arm, and over the top of the shoulder. It then reaches the base of the skull below the ear, up the rear of the ear, loops over the top to the front of the ear then, extends out to end at the outside edge of the eyebrow.

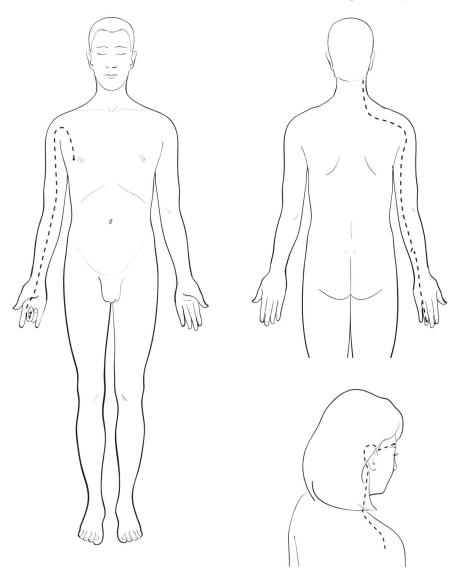

The Gall Bladder Channel

The Gall Bladder channel has 44 points. It begins at the outside edge of the eye, and then loops back over the side of the head to the base of the skull. It then moves down the neck to the top of the shoulder, from where it zigzags in front of the shoulder, down the side of the body to the hip, and down the outside of the leg past the knee to the ankle, ending on the outside nail point of the fourth toe.

The Liver Channel

The Liver channel has 14 points. It begins on the outside nail point of the big toe, ascends up the foot to the ankle, then up the inside of the lower leg, past the knee, and up the inside of the thigh to the crease of the groin. It then descends the crease slightly, moves at an angle across the torso up to the tip of the 11th rib, to end on the edge of the rib cage at a level halfway between the navel and the sternum.

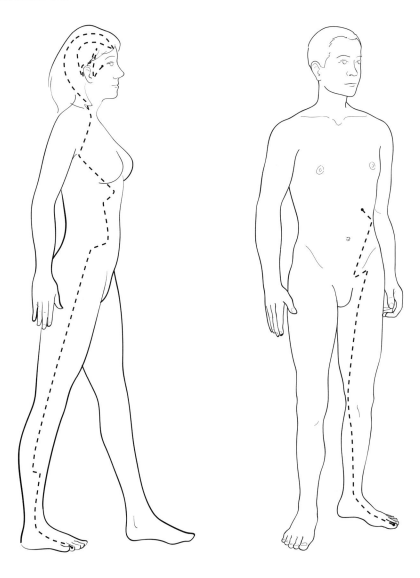

The Lung Channel

The Lung channel has 11 points. It begins in the valley crease where the arm meets the torso, ascends upwards and over the front of the shoulder, then runs down the outside of the inside arm, past the elbow to the wrist, up the base of the thumb to end at the outside nail point of the thumb.

The Colon Channel

The Colon channel has 20 points. It begins on the outside nail point of the index finger, ascends up the finger into the valley between finger and thumb, up the outside of the outside arm, past the elbow and up the upper arm, over the outside shoulder, over the neck and jaw, to end at the side of the nose.

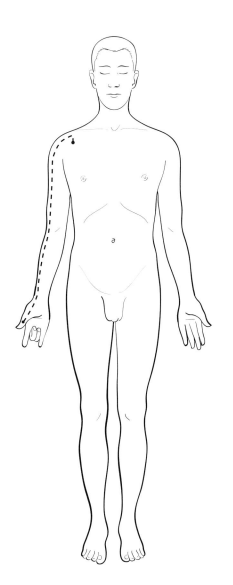

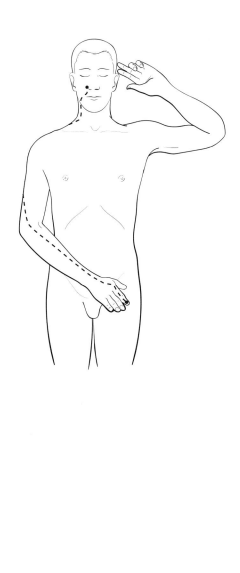

The Stomach Channel

The Stomach channel has 45 points. It begins on the lower edge of the eye socket and moves down the face to the rim of the jaw. From the jaw, the channel descends over the neck to the collarbone, moves outwards to the nipple line, and continues downward over the front of the torso, to the groin. It then moves to the outside of the upper leg, where it continues down to end on the outside nail point of the second toe.

The Spleen Channel

The Spleen channel has 21 points. It begins on the inside nail point of the big toe, ascends along the edge of the toe to the side of the ankle, where it then continues up the lower leg, knee and inside thigh to the groin. It then goes up the front of the torso to the outside of the chest, beneath the front of the shoulder, and angles back down to end on the side of the torso, under the arm.

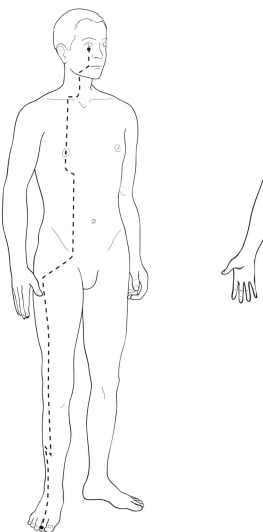

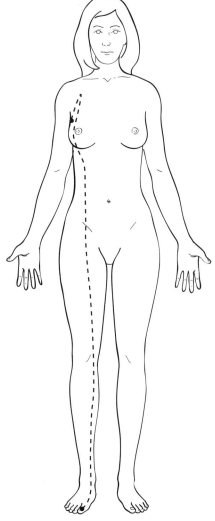

The Eight Extraordinary Meridians

These are also known as the Eight Miraculous Meridians, the Eight Strange Flows, the Eight Miscellaneous Channels, and the Eight Psychic Pathways. These channels are seen as "oceans" of energy—reservoirs that can be drawn upon if there is a deficiency, or to accommodate any excess. The Extraordinary meridians form the basis of the initial stages of Chi Kung practice, and they constitute its main framework. They are in four sets of pairs:

- Governor (Du) and Conception (Ren);
- Thrusting (Chong) and Girdle (Dai);
- Yin Qiao and Yang Qiao;
- Yin Wei and Yang Wei.

(The Chinese word "Mo" means "channel" so, for instance, the Governor channel would be Du Mo.) In an alternative arrangement, the channels are grouped in pairs with a major channel and a support channel, as follows:

- Governor (Du) and Yang Qiao;
- Conception (Ren) and Yin Qiao;
- Girdle (Dai) and Yang Wei;
- Thrusting (Chong) and Yin Wei.

This pairing of these channels is important when considering the Master and Coupled points (*see* page 62). In Chi Kung practice these are not the same as the Acupuncture pathways.

The Eight Extraordinary meridians are said to originate at the very earliest stages of life— in the embryo itself. It has been suggested that they are involved in the initial division of a cell causing it to split into two, then into four cells, then eight. This could be seen as providing the primary framework that makes us what we are—a front and a back, a center line up the middle and a circular belt that surrounds it all.

This may relate to the primary organizing principle known as the Pa Kua—the eight diagrams (*see* page 44). The division into eight patterns is also fundamental to the possible variations of Yin and Yang—as seen in the eight trigrams of the *I Ching*. It has been proposed that the division into eight basic patterns is indeed the basic pattern—the underlying logic— of how everything works. The Eight Extraordinary meridians may be the manifestation of this in ourselves. In Chi Kung they provide the infrastructure of the body-energy system and form the basis of all the major organ channels. They are important because along them are many points of intersection, at which a number of the other primary channels meet together.

A knowledge of these channels is prerequisite to a clear understanding of Chi Kung. It allows a person to look at all forms of Chi Kung and "read" and understand them, just as somebody who knows words, grammar, and syntax can read and understand a report.

Governor Channel/Du Mo

The Governor channel has 28 points. It runs up the center of the back and over the head to end on the top lip. Together with the Conception channel, the Governor channel is fundamental to the first stages of Chi Kung practice in activating and circulating the Microcosmic Orbit. It is supported by:

Yang Qiao Mo

The Yang Qiao Mo which runs from the heel (Qiao) up the side of the body, over the shoulder, up the front of the face and over the head to end at the base of the skull.

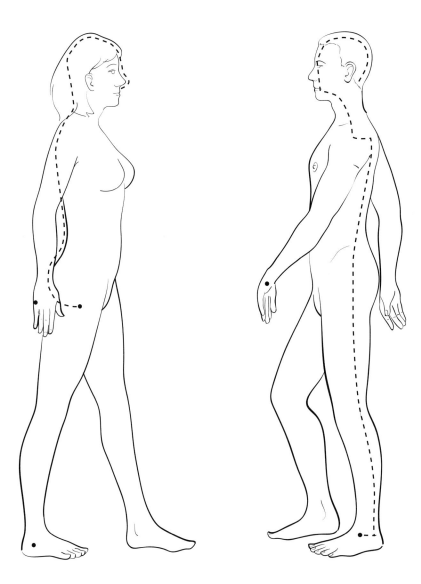

Conception Channel/Ren Mo

The Conception channel has 24 points. It runs up the center of the front, ending on the bottom lip. It is supported by:

Yin Qiao Mo

The Yin Qiao Mo which runs from the inside of the foot, up the inside leg and front of the torso, to the collarbone, over the neck and face to end at the inside corner of the eye.

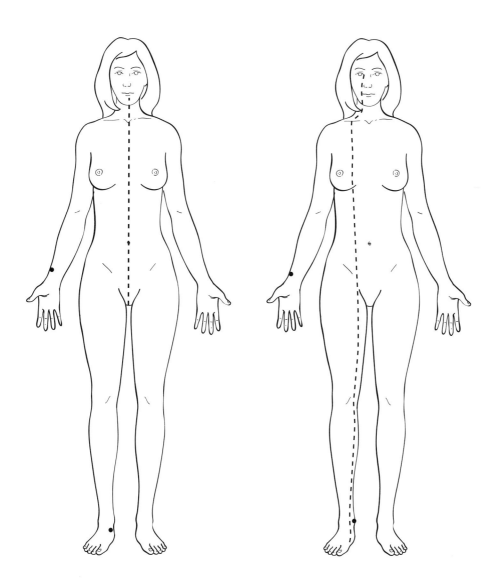

Girdle Channel/Dai Mo

The Girdle channel has no separate points of its own. It is the only channel that runs horizontally around the body—all the others run vertically. In Chi Kung this "belt channel" not only circulates at the waist, but also envelops the whole of the body from top to bottom, and outside of it to the edge of the bio-electromagnetic field, like a cocoon. It is supported by:

Yang Wei Mo

The Yang Wei Mo which runs from the base of the skull, over the head, down to the shoulder and on down the side of the body to end on the foot.

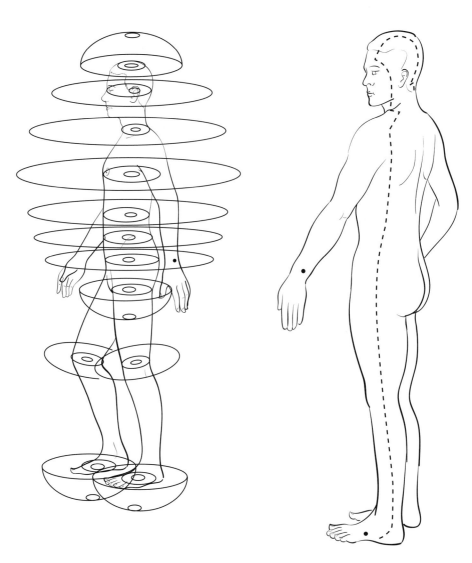

Thrusting Channel/Chong Mo

The Thrusting channel runs directly up the center of the body, from the perineum to the crown. It is about three inches wide and along it are "cauldrons," centers of energy concentration, known in the Yogic tradition as "chakras." These are approximately at the same horizontal level as the related points of the Microcosmic Orbit on the surface of the body on the Governor and Conception channels (*see* page 99). It is supported by:

Yin Wei Mo

The Yin Wei Mo which runs from the top of the throat, down the front of the neck, on down the side of the front torso and inside leg to end on the lower leg.

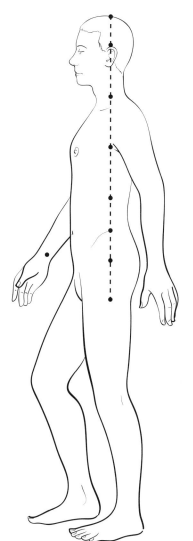

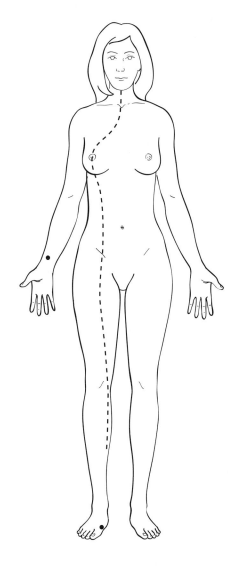

The Twelve Primary Chi Kung Points

These are the major points that are at the center of Chi Kung practice. They could be called the "Chi Kung Points." They are all located on specific channels, and are identified as numbered points along those channels. There are various translations of the names, and for a comparison here, the points are identified from two authoritative source books: The first name given is from *Traditional Chinese Acupuncture, Volume 1, Meridians and Points* by Prof. J.R. Worsley. The second name is from *Acupuncture: A Comprehensive Text*, the textbook of the Shanghai College of Traditional Medicine, translated by John O'Connor and Dan Bensky.

POINT	LOCATION	CHINESE NAME
The Navel	Conception channel 8	Spirit Deficiency/Shenchueh
	Located in the center of the navel	Middle of the Navel/Qizhong
Rear Navel	Governor channel 4	Gate of Life/Ming Men
	On the center line of the back, between the second and third lumbar vertebrae	Life's Door/Mingmen
The Crown	Governor channel 20	One Hundred Meetings/PaiHui
	Middle line of the head, slightly back from the top	Hundred Meetings/Baihui
The Perineum	Conception channel 1	Meeting of Yin/Huiyin
	Midway between the genitals and anus	Perineum/Huiyin
The Palms	Pericardium channel 8	Palace of Weariness/Laokung
	On the palm of the hand, between the third and fourth metacarpal bones on the "head" line crease	Labor's Palace/Laogong
The Soles	Kidney channel 1	Bubbling Spring/Yungchuan
	On the center of the bottom of the foot, between the second and third metatarsal bones, in the crease	Gushing Spring/Yongquan
The Heart	Conception channel 17	Within the Breast/Shanchung
	On the front of the chest, level with the fourth intercostal space/ the nipples on a man	Penetrating Odor/Shanzhong
Rear Heart	Governor channel 11	Spirit Path/Shentao
	On the middle line of the back, between the fifth and sixth thoracic vertebrae	Spirit's Path/Shendao

The Brow	Governor channel 24.5	No name given
	Between the eyebrows	No name given
Tip of Tongue	Not on any regular channel	No name given
	Tip of the tongue	No name given

All these points are commonly used in many Chi Kung practices. There is only one way to learn them, and that is simply to learn them—sometimes there is no substitute for repetitive learning. You will find them invaluable in all future practices.

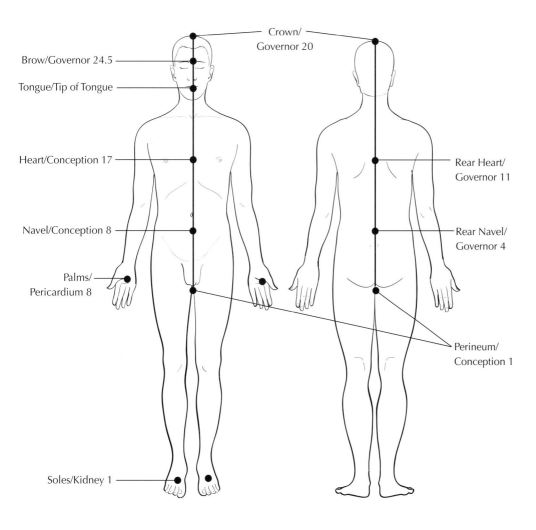

The 12 Primary Chi Kung Points

The Master and Coupled Points

The Master and Coupled points are a special category of points that can be used to access and activate the Eight Extraordinary meridians. Each of the Eight Extraordinary meridians has a Master point and a Coupled point—one on the hand and the other on the foot. Each also has a paired meridian and on the paired meridian the Master and Coupled points are the reverse, so that the Master point of one is the Coupled point of the other, and vice versa, such that there is a reciprocal relationship between the points on each pair of meridians. These sets of paired meridians are as follows:

- Du Mo and Yang Qiao Mo;
- Ren Mo and Yin Qiao Mo;
- Dai Mo and Yang Wei Mo;
- Chong Mo and Yin Wei Mo.

Knowing the location of these points allows you to access and affect the Eight Extraordinary meridians and this is especially useful because there is no easy method for "reading" or diagnosing them. They are not readable on the pulse readings, although they are vaguely reflected on the pulses in that their effect may be observed on the pulses, but cannot be easily or plainly diagnosed. This is a mysterious area of Chi Kung warranting further study, since the Eight Extraordinary channels are so fundamental and important.

The Master and Coupled points are as follows. Again, the names given are first from Prof. J.R. Worsley, followed by those from the Shanghai *Comprehensive Text*.

Du Mo
Small Intestine channel 3
Back Ravine/Back Creek

Yang Qiao Mo
Bladder channel 62
Extended Meridian/Extending Vessel

Ren Mo

Lung channel 7
Narrow Defile/Broken Sequence

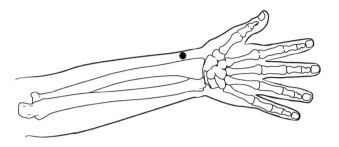

Yin Qiao Mo

Kidney channel 6
Illuminated Sea/Shining Sea

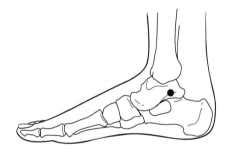

Dai Mo

Gall Bladder channel 41
Foot Above Tears/Near Tears on the Foot

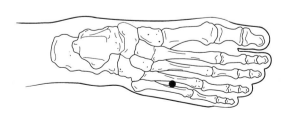

64 Yang Wei Mo
Triple Heater channel 5
Outer Frontier Gate/Outer Gate

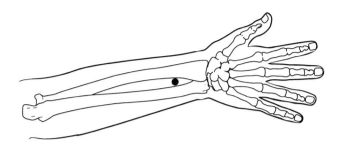

Chong Mo
Spleen channel 4
Prince's Grandson/Grandfather's Grandson

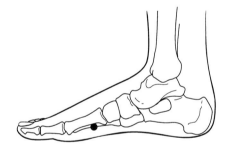

Yin Wei Mo
Pericardium 6
Inner Frontier Gate/Inner Gate

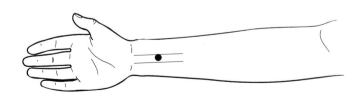

Jing Chi Shen

Jing, Chi, and Shen are the Three Treasures that the Chinese understand to constitute the three basic components of a human being. They are cultivated in the Three Tan T'ien (*see* page 83). In Chi Kung they are often run together into a single word—"JingChiShen."

JING

Jing is the genetic energy inherited from our parents and ancestors, and it is also our sexual energy. It is vital to preserve this, and there are many practices in Chinese sexual manuals for this purpose. Males have Yang Jing and females have Yin Jing, each of which needs aspects of the other to stay balanced and healthy.

CHI

Chi is the energy that we run on. It has many different forms, such as Ta Chi, Ku Chi, Yuan Chi, Jing Chi, and Wei Chi. It can be depleted by overwork, malnourishment, incorrect habits, and too much sex. It is developed, in part, from Jing which provides the foundation for it.

SHEN

Shen is a general term for Consciousness and Spirit. The spirit is fed and nourished by the Chi. The spirit body is of a higher level or frequency than the Chi and it is dependent on it. It is said to reside in the heart, and a person's Shen can easily be seen in their eyes. Someone with good Shen has eyes that sparkle and are alive, while a person with poor Shen has dull eyes that seem to be covered over and hidden.

The relationship between Jin, Chi, and Shen may be compared with the recently adopted Western term of Mind, Body, and Spirit. However, the Western version, while attempting to reunite these three components, may miss the point because it does not incorporate a comprehensive understanding of the biological reality of our energy system—our essence, energy, and spirit.

Jing, Chi, and Shen are hierarchically based on each other, and there are things we can do to preserve, nourish, and cultivate them, and also things which will empty, deplete, and undermine them. A Chi Kung practitioner's actions, habits, and practices are largely based upon and determined by whatever will increase or decrease Jing, Chi, and Shen. They are, indeed, our most precious and valuable possessions.

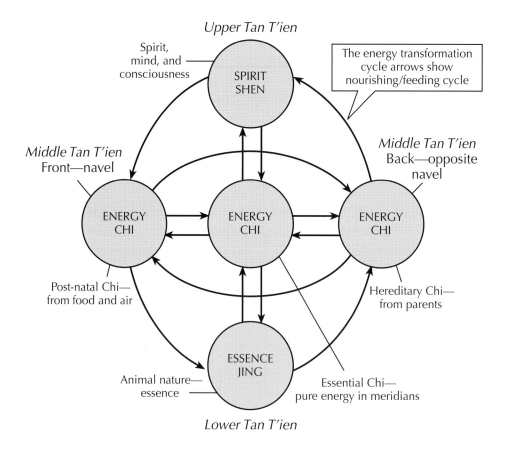

Upper Tan T'ien

Spirit, mind, and consciousness

SPIRIT SHEN

The energy transformation cycle arrows show nourishing/feeding cycle

Middle Tan T'ien Front—navel

Middle Tan T'ien Back—opposite navel

ENERGY CHI

ENERGY CHI

ENERGY CHI

Post-natal Chi— from food and air

Hereditary Chi— from parents

ESSENCE JING

Animal nature— essence

Essential Chi— pure energy in meridians

Lower Tan T'ien

The Three Treasures and their Transformations—Essence, Energy, Spirit—Jing, Chi, Shen

An Overview of the Channels and Pathways

The twelve major organ channels and the Eight Extraordinary meridians together constitute a comprehensive and integrated energy system for the body. When they are open and working properly, the system is fully functioning and will regulate itself automatically, so that the Chi flows how and where it should. It will regulate itself in response to the daily circulation, the Moon cycle, and the annual cycle of the seasons. It will respond appropriately to external events, and the emotions and feelings will be in order and available. Your energy will function as it is intended to.

To appreciate this system as an integrated whole, rather than just a collection of individual meridians and points, it may be helpful to look at one particular circulation—the Wei circulation (the surface circulation). It follows a specific sequence, as follows:

Heart begins on the torso and flows down the inside arm to the hand. This flows into:

Small Intestine, which begins on the hand and flows up the outside arm to the head. Then:

Bladder, which begins at the corner of the eye and flows up and over the head then down the back to the feet. This flows into:

Kidneys, which begins on the bottom of the feet and flows up the inside leg and front of the torso to end at the top of the chest.

Overall, the circulation can be summarized as having four sections—chest, hand, head, foot, and back to the chest. As there are twelve organ channels, this circulation is repeated twice more. To continue:

Pericardium, follows on from the kidneys and flows again down the inside arm to the hands. This flows into:

Triple Heater, runs up the outside arm to the head and outside of the eyebrow. Then:

Gall Bladder, which begins at the outside corner of the eye, over the side of the head, down the side of the body, to end on the feet. This flows into:

Liver, which begins at the big toe, flows up the inside leg to the lower abdomen and continues across the front of the body to end on the side of the rib cage.

One final circulation follows.

Lungs, begins on the torso, runs down the inside arms to the hands. This flows into:

Colon, which flows from the hands, up the arms and over the shoulders to the point on the side of the nose. This flows into:

Stomach, which begins below the eye, runs down the face and over the front of the chest and torso, then down the outside legs to end on the feet. This flows into:

Spleen, which begins on the big toe, then runs up the inside leg and up the torso to end on the side of the chest.

This then flows back into the **Heart**, thus completing the whole circuit.

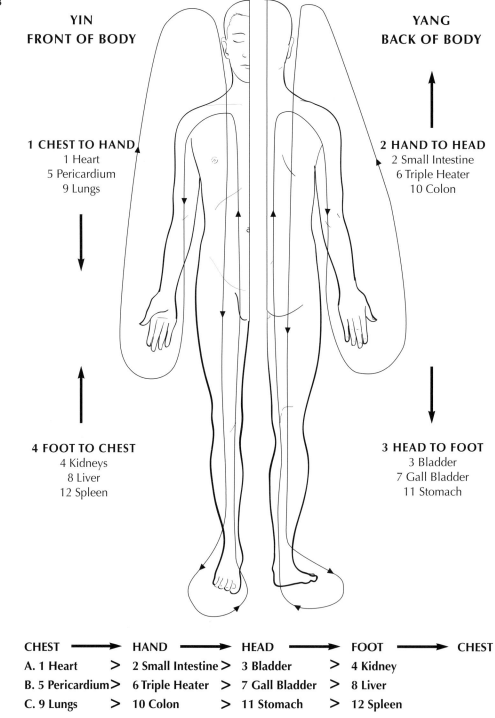

YIN
FRONT OF BODY

YANG
BACK OF BODY

1 CHEST TO HAND
1 Heart
5 Pericardium
9 Lungs

2 HAND TO HEAD
2 Small Intestine
6 Triple Heater
10 Colon

4 FOOT TO CHEST
4 Kidneys
8 Liver
12 Spleen

3 HEAD TO FOOT
3 Bladder
7 Gall Bladder
11 Stomach

CHEST →	HAND →	HEAD →	FOOT →	CHEST
A. 1 Heart >	**2 Small Intestine** >	**3 Bladder** >	**4 Kidney**	
B. 5 Pericardium >	**6 Triple Heater** >	**7 Gall Bladder** >	**8 Liver**	
C. 9 Lungs >	**10 Colon** >	**11 Stomach** >	**12 Spleen**	

Overview of Channels and Pathways

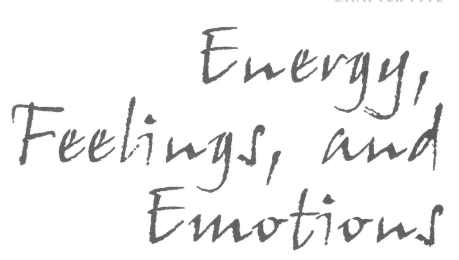

CHAPTER FIVE

氣功

Energy, Feelings, and Emotions

The Chi Kung of Feelings and Emotions

Feelings and emotions are our experience of different states of being within ourselves. In the West this has now become mainly the province of psychology, psychiatry, and psychotherapy. One of the most remarkable aspects of these fields is that there is no consensus as to what our emotions are or how they function, only a range of opinions and theoretical models.

Although they are often translated as Wants, Needs, Desires, and such we are still not sure what emotions and feelings are. From a Chi Kung standpoint this is because we do not take into account the reality of the energy system, and this is like trying to play a game without knowing all of the rules.

THE FIVE ELEMENTS AND THE EMOTIONS

In Chi Kung, the relationship between the emotions and the energy system is firmly established. Again this relates to the Five Elements theory. Each of the Elements of Wood, Fire, Earth, Metal, and Water relates to specific internal organs. These Elements are also related to the seasons of Spring, Summer, Late-Summer, Fall, and Winter, created by the rotation of the Earth around the Sun. The qualities, characteristics, and power of each season are reflected in each Element and their related organs (*see* the Table of Correspondences, page 40).

These qualities each have positive and negative aspects—whether they are ideally balanced and in harmonious relationship with everything else, or whether they are Excessive or Deficient, Yang or Yin. In this context, both excess and deficiency are detrimental and undesirable. The greater the deviation from a natural balance in the organs, the more distorted and out of balance the particular emotions will be. Emotional health occurs when the energy functions correctly in the organs.

Certain words in the English language have come to describe the emotions and how they relate to the Elements. However, these translations of the Chinese terms do not do justice to, or adequately describe, the totality of the original meanings. Therefore, I am adding my own variations to describe both the positive and negative dimensions of these words. The commonly accepted word appears first, with its counter-balancing word following:

WOOD	Liver and Gall Bladder	Anger/Power
FIRE	Heart, Small Intestines, Pericardium and Triple Heater	Joy/Anxiety
EARTH	Spleen and Stomach	Sympathy/Worry
METAL	Lungs and Colon	Grief/Purification
WATER	Kidneys and Bladder	Fear/Awe

In an Inner Alchemy practice called The Fusion of the Five Elements, the negative energy in each organ is cleansed, purified, and broken down into its harmless basic constituents—just as a poison can be broken into its constituent substances and lose its harmful effect. The emotions are then neutralized and brought back into center, balance, and harmony. It may be that our emotions are simply indicators of the energy experience we are having.

From this perspective, emotions are not desirable—either in excess or deficiency—because they drain energy out of a person. It is best to exist in neutral, in the center place, ready and able to respond in the appropriate manner to any given situation. This may explain why Chinese and other Eastern cultures are reputed to be "inscrutable." Quite simply, they may be working hard not to feel, but to stay in center. In the West we may have our emotional priorities wrong.

In the Inner Alchemy tradition, when the art of living beyond one's emotions has been achieved, there is a progression toward the cultivation of the Virtues. As with emotions, virtues are related to the internal foundation of the Five Elements and the five organs/officials. Each organ/official has a higher level of itself, which is achieved when it is functioning at its best. This is its Virtue. Inner Alchemy practice cultivates these Virtues, as follows:

Liver and Gall Bladder	Kindness
Heart, Small Intestine, Pericardium and Triple Heater	Honor and Respect
Spleen and Stomach	Fairness
Lungs and Colon	Righteousness
Kidneys and Bladder	Gentleness

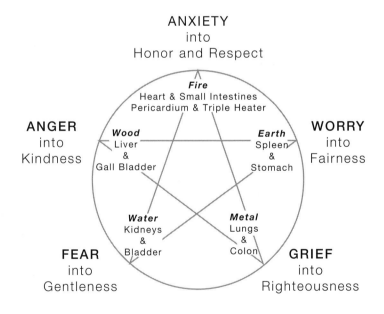

Sum Total of the Virtues = Goodness

The Transformation of Negative Emotions through the Five Elements and the Cultivation of the Virtues

Combine all of these virtues together and the sum total, the point to aim for, is Goodness. The emotions and feelings are based on the healthy functioning of our internal organs/officials, which in turn is based on having one's energy system working correctly. So, to be emotionally healthy you have to be energetically healthy—balanced and free-flowing with the right quality, good volume, and correct relationships.

If you are feeling depressed, unhappy, worried, sad, or fearful, it is necessary to put your energy right, through self-practice or with a practitioner, and then the unwanted emotions and feelings will diminish or disappear altogether.

Other Energy Systems

Clearly, there are a wide range of possible applications of Chi Kung, each with its own merits, strengths, and appropriate uses. In fact, the possibilities are so diverse that it may seem that Chi Kung is all that you have to do. However, Chi Kung has grown within the context of the Chinese and Asian traditions and it is only one of several ways of understanding how our energy works.

One of the reasons that there is no tradition equivalent to Chi Kung in the West is that we have had no model of energy similar to the meridian system. However, the meridian system is not the complete, nor the only, picture of energy in the body. Other cultures have developed parallel systems, and they each have their own practices and traditions. There are many body-energy practices and manifestations in Western history and culture, although there are rarely explanations of how the energy system operates.

In each, there is a clear distinction between the "gross anatomy" (what we can see and feel—the flesh, blood, and bones) and the "energy anatomy" (that we cannot see and feel). This latter has come to be called the "subtle anatomy" or "energy-body." This is the missing chapter of *Gray's Anatomy*—the anatomical textbook that is the bible of Western medical science. Without the energy-body many things do not make sense. Include the energy-body in the picture and suddenly everything begins to fit together into one coherent whole.

COMPARATIVE BODY-ENERGY SYSTEMS

There are three major body-energy models. They are separate and distinct, but they do overlap and cover some of the same ground. Each one consists of a complete body of knowledge, with its own paradigms and parameters. Each has its own complete and independent anatomy and physiology. They have become known and identified by the following names:

- The Meridian System;
- The Chakra System;
- The Aura Field.

These three body-energy models are the basic framework by which body-energy functions and each of them is the basis and the ground for all kinds of methods, techniques, and practices.

The Meridian System

The meridian system is the foundation of Chi Kung practice, and it is also the basis of Oriental medicine, martial arts, and a tradition of spiritual development. The main features of this system are:

- There are 12 major meridians, each related to a particular organ.
- There are Eight Extraordinary meridians which are reservoirs of energy.
- There is an energy field, the Wei Chi, that extends outside and around the body, but it is not very differentiated.
- There is a spectrum of relationships and correspondences between meridians, organs, tissues, sense organs, and emotional and mental facilities.
- There are three levels of energy—Jing, Chi, and Shen.
- There are three energy centers—the lower, middle, and upper Tan T'ien.
- Cultivation of the energy provides the foundation for development of the Soul and Spirit.

The Chakra System

The Chakras are the central element and main focus of Indian spiritual and religious traditions, such as Hinduism and Buddhism, and they are at the core of the practices of Yoga and Ayurveda. Like the Taoists, Yogis are known for their extraordinary abilities and their spiritual development, and these are based primarily on their control of energy. In many ways Chi Kung and Yoga are equivalent in their respective cultural traditions. The main features of this system are:

- There are seven major Chakras.
- Each Chakra has a name and a specific location.
- Each Chakra has an associated endocrine gland.
- Each Chakra has a related organ(s) and area of the body.
- Each Chakra has emotional and psychological characteristics.
- There is an ascending hierarchy of functions.
- The Chakras relate to the Soul and the Spirit.

The Chakra system is at the foundation of yogic practice and the spiritual traditions of India. It is a separate, independent, and self-contained body-energy model, with its own range of methods and applications. Its use pre-dates recorded history.

The Aura Field

The Aura Field is the energy field that flows outside and around the body. Knowledge of this field is highly developed in the Western esoteric tradition, and it is also deeply integrated in the Indian model. There is, however, little correspondence to the Oriental meridian model. In terms of the anatomy and physiology of the Aura there is basic common agreement about certain things:

- **There are seven different energy field levels.**
- **The fields are of increasingly higher and more refined frequency.**
- **The fields relate to each other in a series of harmonics.**
- **Each field has a specific color, which reflects its state of functioning.**
- **The fields have an ascending hierarchical relationship to each other.**
- **The fields interact with the Chakras.**
- **The higher fields are related to what we describe as the Soul and the Spirit.**

The Aura extends out around the body like an antenna, and it is through this that external energies and influences primarily are able to affect our bodies.

THE ENERGY BODY

Each of these energy body models developed independently, in the context of its own culture. Each is essentially complete, but no single one is the whole story. However, when you put them together, and overlay them over each other, you then have a complete picture of the energy body. Perhaps we are now moving toward an explanation and understanding of the relationships and interactions between the three models and how they constitute the energy body. Our having a healthy energy body is clearly fundamental to our individual and collective well-being, and it is the emerging definition of the state of our health.

CONTEMPORARY ECLECTIC

In addition to the more traditional methods and techniques of working with body-energy, there has been a surge of new developments over the last few years. These have grown out of the natural medicine and holistic health movement. There are many of these new techniques and therapies, and they include: Energy Balancing, Biokinesiology, Psycho-Physical Therapies,

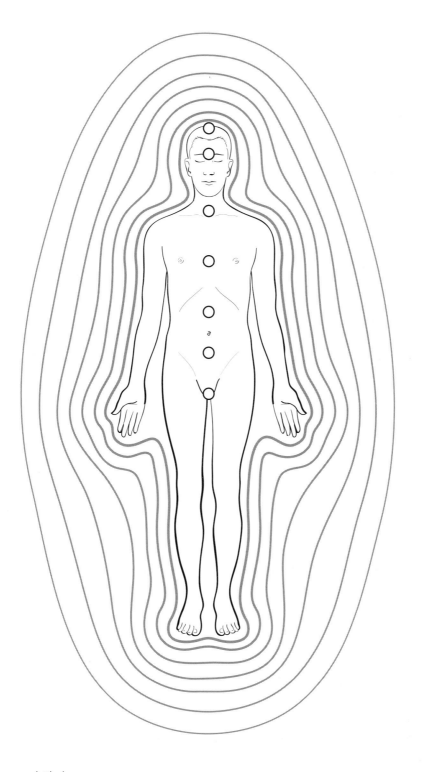

The Aura and Chakras

Bio-Energetics, Core Energetics, Body-Centered Psychotherapy, Healing Touch, Touch For Health, Therapeutic Touch, and Energy Healing.

Some of these are excellent, some are not, and a great deal depends on the experience, skill, and ability of the practitioner in question. Use your own judgment and intuition, as well as your experience and response, as the guide when trying any of these techniques or a particular practitioner.

Therapeutic Touch

Therapeutic Touch is one recent system which has grown in the US under scientific scrutiny, and which in many ways is the Western equivalent of Chi Kung. It is now widely accepted and integrated into Western medical science and is now approved for use by nurses in hospitals and other clinical settings. Just as Chi Kung has been called "Chinese Therapeutic Touch," then Therapeutic Touch could be called "Western Chi Kung."

Therapeutic Touch is both a medical science and a healing art. It is the name given to a broad range of hands-on healing techniques and it incorporates many ancient and modern methods of healing which involve passing energy from a healer to an individual. The techniques include such methods as Aura Clearing, Centering, Chakra Balancing, Focusing, Healing Rituals, and Trauma Release. The title "Nurse Healer" has come to be used for these practitioners.

Another important aspect is that it is not limited to use in a professional context; it is equally available to the layperson. It can be learnt and applied by anybody who is prepared to undergo the necessary training. Everyone is a healer. Mothers can use it for their children; couples can do it to each other; friends can use it as a caring and giving activity together; you can even use it to take care of your pets.

Therapeutic Touch and Chi Kung Healing

Obviously Therapeutic Touch has great affinities with Chi Kung Healing. There are a lot of similarities in approach and technique. While Chi Kung healers have an established model of anatomy and physiology in the meridian system, Western healers and Therapeutic Touch practitioners have developed from a more intuitive and experiential approach. Having said this, Chi Kung practitioners could probably make perfect sense of the work of Therapeutic Touch practitioners, and vice versa.

PART THREE

Activating Your Energy

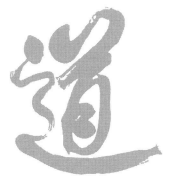

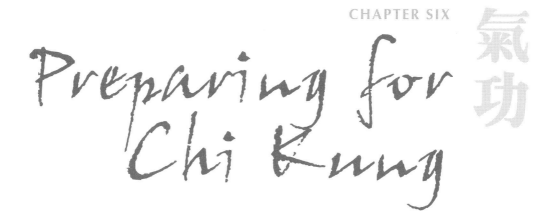

CHAPTER SIX

Preparing for Chi Kung

氣功

Your Attitude and Approach

In order to practice Chi Kung you will need to be prepared on a mental as well as a physical level. It is most important to have the correct attitude and approach, as your beliefs and attitude are as significant as what you do physically.

PREPARATION AND WARM-UP

To begin to practice Chi Kung you first need to prepare, just as you would before doing physical exercises. You will need to get ready in a number of ways:

- **Preparing your time;**
- **Preparing your environment;**
- **Preparing your mind;**
- **Preparing your breathing;**
- **Preparing your body.**

Preparing your time

The only way that you can do Chi Kung is to set aside time. Consider this as special time for yourself—like a gift, taking a vacation, or a reward. Imagine that you are going to a particular place, such as a health club to work out, and nothing will interrupt you. This can be for five minutes or the whole day. Just make sure that you will not be disturbed or distracted, because you are entering into an internalized meditative state and you need to stay focused. This is a sacred time.

Preparing your environment

Your environment is where you happen to be at any given time—this may be in the familiar surroundings of your home, or in a garden, park, gymnasium, or public space. The choice is entirely up to you, but unless you have developed great control over your concentration, a parking lot in a busy shopping center on a Saturday afternoon would not be an ideal environment. You may practice alone, with a partner, in a small group, or in a massed gathering. Do whatever you can to select an environment conducive to practice, and with the best natural Chi. Eliminate possible distractions, and, if all else fails, you can always be assured of 15 minutes of complete uninterrupted privacy in your own bathroom!

Preparing your mind

There are many ways to prepare your mind, a number of which are described and incorporated in practice sequences in this book. However, in mental preparation there are essential elements common to all forms. Keep your mind clear. Do not get distracted by other thoughts. Stay focused on the awareness of your internal experience. Be empty, like a blank page. Be prepared to accept and recognize whatever your experience is. Imagine that it will be like opening a package and you do not know what is inside it. Allow it to be a surprise!

Preparing your breathing

Breathing has two aspects—unconscious and conscious. Your breathing happens automatically, it is a primary function, and you do not need to be aware of it for it to take place. However, you can consciously and purposefully adjust your breathing by paying attention to it. You can slow it down or speed it up. You can take deep slow breaths or short fast ones. Make sure that you are not constricted at the waist, because this will inhibit the ability of your diaphragm to descend and draw air in to your lungs. Simply placing your attention on your breathing is one of the fastest ways of centering inside yourself.

Preparing your body

Your physical body is where your energy resides and circulates. It has been described as the temple of your Spirit and Soul. Our physical bodies have evolved over ages out of the material of the universe. We are the structure of the whole of creation, as reflected in the saying "As Above, So Below." We each contain and reflect the innate structure of everything else and are each a microcosm of the macrocosm. Stay aware of this simple fact as you prepare to practice. Before you start, it is best to be rested. Attend to any natural functions before beginning practice. Maybe take a shower or bath so that you feel clean and fresh. Wear loose, comfortable clothes.

Preparing your time, environment, mind, breathing, and body will provide you with the optimum context to begin to practice—and to get the Chi.

THE AWAKENED MIND

When you enter into the Chi Kung state, be aware that there is a corresponding change in your brainwaves. You are literally changing your mind and your state of consciousness. The four major brainwaves are in ranges of frequencies across a continuous spectrum. These rhythms are known as Beta (38–16 cycles per second), Alpha (15–9 cps), Theta (8–4 cps), and Delta (3–0.5 cps).

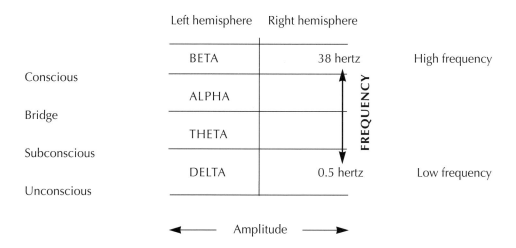

Brainwave Patterns

- **Beta rhythms are the highest frequencies and are involved in the use of words, language, analysis, and logical thinking. They scan at a fast speed. For most people this is identified as the act of thinking.**
- **Alpha rhythms control and generate a state of calm, detached awareness. This is the gateway to meditation and the Chi Kung state.**

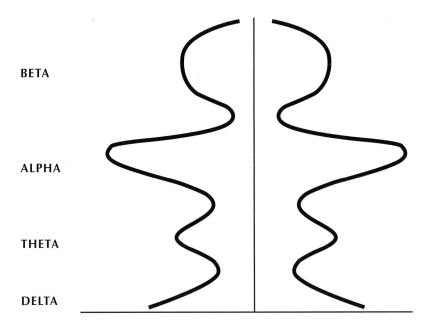

BETA

ALPHA

THETA

DELTA

The Awakened Mind Pattern

- Theta rhythms relate to the subconscious mind, the vast part of your consciousness that you are usually unaware of. This corresponds to dreams, myths, inner impulses, depth of insight, and profundity.
- Delta rhythms are the slowest and they relate to the unconscious. It is experienced in deep sleep. This is the maintenance level of the basic functions at our primary biological level.

When you begin to practice, consciously or otherwise, you decrease Beta ("thinking") brainwaves, and increase Alpha brainwaves, so inducing a state of calm, detached awareness. You enter into the Chi Kung state.

Healers, swamis, and those in heightened states of awareness have been identified as generating specific brainwave patterns—the relationship between Beta, Alpha, Theta, and Delta— described as the optimal state of consciousness. This leads to what has been called the "High Performance Mind" or the "Awakened Mind."

Meditation in Chi Kung

In those Chi cultivation disciplines that have become known as Chi Kung it is traditional to refer to the "Three Regulations"—the regulation of the body, the breath, and the mind. Chi Kung always involves the regulation of the mind. This is often referred to as meditation and it is why Tai Chi is called a moving meditation. Many forms of Chi Kung, such as Quiescent Chi Kung or Meditative Chi Kung, have no body movement, and they focus primarily on meditation. This is also known as Nei Dan (Internal Chi Kung).

There are two aspects to Chi Kung meditation. The first is to relax completely in a state of full alertness and awareness. Relaxation without awareness is sleep. Much of the physiological benefit of Chi Kung is based on the results of alert relaxation within the human system. This is known as the "Relaxation Response." The second aspect is what the Chinese call "Mind Intent." With mind intent the Chi Kung practitioner purposefully leads or directs the Chi to the organs or glands, circulates the Chi to particular body regions, and induces the flow of Chi in the meridians. There are entire Chi Kung forms based on the use of mind intent to direct Chi. The infusion of universal energy in the form of the Five Elements into the Five Primary Organs—the heart, spleen, lungs, kidneys, and liver—is a classic form of Chi Kung meditation. The induction of the flow of Chi in the Eight Extraordinary meridians is yet another Chi Kung meditation (*see* page 55).

Meditation quickens, nourishes, accelerates, and optimizes the Chi by removing any influences that neutralize its potential efficacy. It is said that when the mind is busy or distracted then the Chi scatters. Meditation relaxes the nervous system and creates the capacity for exercising the key to Chi Kung—mind intent.

THE THREE TAN T'IEN MEDITATION

There are hundreds of Chi Kung meditations. One of the most basic and common is called the Three Tan T'ien meditation. Tan T'ien is best translated as "Elixir Field" (*see also* page 21). Elixir is a highly refined medicine, and Field is a location. The Three Tan T'ien are located as follows:

- **the lower is just below the umbilicus (ovaries, prostate, and lower abdomen);**
- **the middle is at the level of the heart (also thymus gland);**
- **the upper is between the eyes (brain, pituitary, pineal, and hypothalamus).**

Each of these areas of the body produces healing resources including hormones, enzymes, and neurotransmitters. This meditation is a powerful exercise in the use of mind intent to maximize the inner elixir.

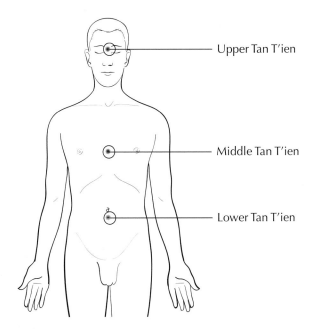

The Three Tan T'ien

Preparation

Find a quiet location where there are few distractions. Sit, lie, or stand comfortably. Deepen and lengthen the breath. Clear your mind. Focus inside yourself. Then begin the Three Tan T'ien practice. Hold your focus at each Tan T'ien until you feel complete.

Lower Tan T'ien

Bring your attention to the area about three finger widths below your navel. Draw both hands up in front of you so they are facing this point, such that the Laokung points (Palace of Weariness) at the center of the palms are radiating toward it. Feel or imagine that your Chi is focused here. Affirm to yourself that this practice causes and enhances activity in the abdominal organs, glands, and tissues, and that it refines a profound internal elixir that heals and empowers your body, mind, and spirit. Now use the mind to open the lower Tan T'ien to the Earth, pull in the energy and vitality of the Earth to mix with the body-energy.

Middle Tan T'ien

Bring your attention to the area around your heart. Draw both hands up so they are facing this point, with the points on the palms radiating toward it. Feel that the Chi from your whole body is focused around your heart and is causing effective activity in the organs, glands, and tissues of the chest including the heart, lungs, and thymus gland. Now use the mind to open the middle Tan T'ien to the biological life of the world. Pull in the energy, vitality, and message of all life forms—plants and animals into the Tan T'ien to mix with the body energy.

Upper Tan T'ien

Now bring your attention to the point between the eyebrows. Draw both hands up so they are facing this point, with the points in the center of the palms radiating toward it. Feel or imagine that the Chi is focused there and is causing effective activity in the organs, glands, and tissues of the head including the brain, pituitary gland, pineal gland, hypothalamus, cerebrospinal fluid system, and the sensory systems of sight, hearing, smell, and taste. Now use the mind to open the upper Tan T'ien to the heavens, to the endless sky and cosmos. Pull in the energy, vitality, and message of all celestial forces—the planets, stars, and space—to mix with the body-energy. Affirm that the upper Tan T'ien is associated with all of the radiance and transcendence of Heaven.

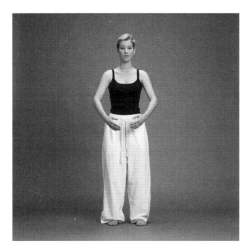

Lower Tan T'ien

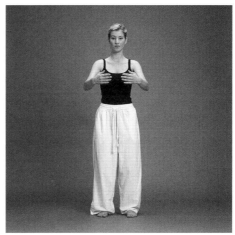

Middle Tan T'ien

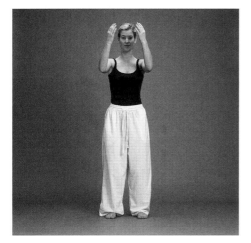

Upper Tan T'ien

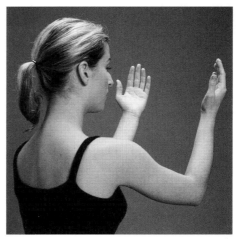

Upper Tan T'ien

On Completion

Take it slowly when re-associating with your local self and your daily associations. Your breath will have found a natural rhythm. Now take a few breaths to re-connect with this day, this time, this location. Do not rush off into the multitude of things you have to do. Take a few moments to integrate the benefits of this practice with your worldly life. Say to yourself something like, "I will take this sense of coordination of my lower, middle, and upper self, and the elixirs of my lower, middle, and upper Tan T'iens into my day, my relationships, and my interactions."

Breathing

Natural, whole-body breathing lies at the heart of Chi Kung. When we breathe with our whole body, as we were designed to do, our breath has a beneficial impact on our physical, emotional, mental, and spiritual health. We feel a sense of energetic wholeness, a sense of being connected to ourselves, to others, and to the environment. When we breathe only in a small part of ourselves, we lose this sense of wholeness, and in so doing we open ourselves up to increasing levels of stress, and we undermine our health and well-being.

Our breath, like our life, is a miracle. Our first breath on Earth began with a cry—with an exhalation, not an inhalation. When we are able to exhale fully, to let go of the old air in our lungs, the inhalation arises as a natural reflex that engages our whole body. That is why Taoist masters remind us to "exhale the old" before we "inhale the new."

Our breath is designed to respond to the changing physical, emotional, mental, and spiritual conditions of our lives. Most of us have noticed how our breathing becomes slower, deeper, and smoother when we experience emotions such as love, happiness, and joy, and how it becomes faster, shallower, and choppier with emotions such as fear, worry, and anger. The speed, depth, and rhythm of our breathing not only reveals a great deal about what is happening inside us, but it also has a powerful influence on our mind and body.

Although some textbooks tell us that the "average" resting adult breath rate is 12–15 times a minute, this is faster than it needs to be. Most of us are so filled with unnecessary physical, emotional, and mental tension that we breathe faster just to supply the extra energy needed to maintain this tension. In contrast, practitioners of Chi Kung and natural, whole-body breathing, experience deep levels of relaxation as well as a dramatic drop in their breathing rate.

The first step in natural breathing is to observe how we actually breathe now, including the internal tensions and imbalances that inhibit our breath. To begin this process we must experience the inter-relationships of the diaphragm, rib cage, and belly.

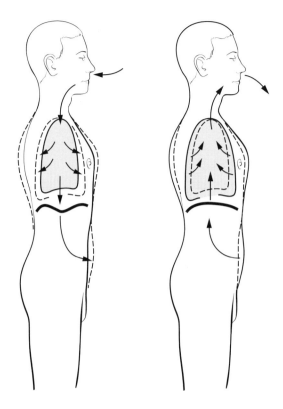

The Direction of Air Flow and the Natural Movement of the Diaphragm When We Breathe

1 The diaphragm is shaped like a dome and it functions as the floor of the chest cavity and the ceiling of the abdominal cavity. It is attached all around the inside of the lower ribs, as well as to the lower lumbar vertebrae.
2 In natural breathing, the diaphragm contracts downward during inhalation and the rib cage expands outward, rising slightly upward, and the belly expands outward. These combined movements create space in the chest cavity for the lungs to expand and take in more air.
3 During exhalation, this movement is reversed as the diaphragm relaxes upward; the combined actions squeeze most of the old air from the lungs.

When the diaphragm, rib cage, and belly can move freely through their full range of motion, we breathe optimally with the least expenditure of effort and energy. What is more, the free up-and-down movement of the diaphragm and gentle bellows-like movements of the rib cage and belly, massage and detoxify our internal organs, help us fight illness, and calm our nerves. Unnecessary tension inhibits the movement of these structures and reduces the amount of air that we exhale and inhale with each breath. To compensate, we often lift our

PREPARING
FOR CHI KUNG

shoulders, breathe mainly in our upper chest, and breathe faster and through our mouth. This can cause us to lose carbon dioxide too quickly which has the effect of constricting our arteries, reducing the amount of oxygen reaching our cells, so propelling us into a state of chronic hyperventilation, making us tense, anxious, irritable, and impatient.

The following exercise, which should be practiced daily, is designed to slow down your breathing and allow it to engage more of yourself.

Practice—Transforming your Breathing

Sit or stand quietly. Sense your weight being supported by the Earth. Follow your breathing as you inhale and exhale through your nose. During inhalation, sense the temperature and vibration of the air as it flows from the tip of your nose through your nasal passages, throat, and trachea on its way into your lungs. During exhalation, sense the air going out of your lungs through your trachea, throat, and nose.

After several minutes, rub your hands together until they are warm and then rest them on your belly. How does your breathing respond to the warmth and energy from your hands? Can you sense the movement and energy of your breath reaching into your belly? Continue following your breathing into and out of your lungs, and notice if your belly expands as you inhale and flattens as you exhale. If your belly does not move easily, see if you can sense what is holding it back. Then use your hands to gently massage your belly. Notice how your breathing now begins to expand into your belly.

Now, with each breath, explore what it means to "exhale the old" and "inhale the new." Release any tensions, worries, and expectations with each exhalation. Sense the fresh, pure energy that enters with each inhalation, using your awareness to guide the energy deep into your belly. Watch, sense, and feel everything that's taking place. Notice how your breath slows down and engages more of yourself.

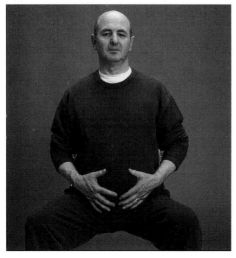

Hands on Belly to Feel your Breathing

CHAPTER SEVEN

Beginning Practices

氣功

What follows is a series of beginning practices that activate your energy system, together with notes on normal activities such as lying and standing. Performing these practices and paying attention to these activities will give you an experience of how your energy feels when it is turned on, moving, and circulating. These directions are general guidelines for getting started. They may be performed in various ways and at different levels of intensity. Begin slowly at first until you get the feel of it, and then vary the degree of concentration and focus according to your level of comfort. They may also be performed in sequence.

The Healing Smile

This is an internal Nei Dan exercise. It is intended to relax and prepare your internal yin organs for practice, calm the mind, and stabilize the metabolism.

1   Find a comfortable position, sitting on a chair with both feet flat on the floor, knees shoulder-width apart, and relax. Clasp your hands in front of you in your lap, with the right over the left, to seal in your Chi. This exercise can also be performed lying down. In this case, clasp your hands and let them rest on your abdomen.

2   Close your eyes. If thoughts appear in your mind, gently let them go and then bring your attention back inside yourself. Pay attention to how you feel.

3   Find a thought, memory, image, or picture that causes you to smile—one of those warm smiles that softens the corners of the mouth.

4   Let the warm, gentle energy of this smile grow and accumulate.

5   Your energy follows your mind. Using your mind bring this smiling energy to the point on your forehead between your eyes, and allow it to accumulate there, like warm water slowly filling a deep bowl.

6   Connect the tip of your tongue with the roof of your mouth, just behind the top of your teeth. This lets the energy flow through your tongue and throat into your torso. In each organ you can hold the healing energy of your smile for as long as you wish, or for the count of a certain number of breaths, or until you feel it overflow. This is indicated by the instruction "Hold your Chi there."

7   Directing the energy with your mind, send this warm, smiling, loving energy to your heart. Let your heart fill with smiling energy. Hold your Chi there.

8   Now send your smiling energy to your lungs. Let your lungs fill with smiling energy. Hold your Chi there.

10 Now send your warm, smiling, healing energy to your liver. Your liver is the largest organ in your body and is situated below your rib cage on your right-hand side. Let your liver fill with smiling, loving energy. Hold your Chi there.

11 Now send your energy to your kidneys. Your kidneys are located halfway between the bottom of your rib cage and the top of your pelvis, level with your waist. They are about the size of clenched fists and are either side of the spine, about one third in from your back. Hold your Chi there.

12 Now send your warm, gentle, loving Chi to your spleen. Your spleen is on the left-hand side of the body, just below the rib cage, opposite your liver. Hold your Chi there.

13 Finally, send your Chi to your navel. When it is at your navel, let go of your smile from the corners of your mouth, so that your mouth is relaxed and neutral, and bring your warm current of smiling energy through one organ after the other—your heart, lungs, liver, kidneys, and spleen—slowly winding it in until it all comes to rest in your navel.

14 If you are male, place the center of your left palm over your navel, then cover it with the center of your right palm. If you are female, place your right palm over your navel and cover it with your left. Stay in this position and feel the warm energy in your navel. This is your Chi and it is now in your Center. Concentrate on feeling and experiencing it there.

15 Pay attention to how you feel, and find a word, phrase, image, or symbol to describe it. Remember this—it is your personal internal "key" to your Chi.

16 Relax your hands and let them take any comfortable position, and slowly open your eyes, one eyelash after the other, and return back to the outside.

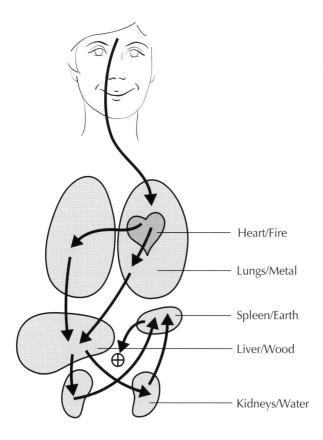

The Healing Smile

You have now smiled at your main internal organs. This simple process is a way of sending your own warm, gentle, loving energy to yourself. It releases tension and stress, and it generates deep relaxation. It calms your emotions, refreshes your sense organs, and stimulates the tissues. It also makes you feel good. Learn this exercise and you can use it whenever you wish. Smile, please!

The Energy Shower

The Energy Shower is an external, Wei Dan exercise. It is an exercise to cleanse negative energy from the major front, middle, and back meridians, to prepare the meridians for further practice, and to bring fresh Chi into you from the outside.

Clearing the Front Channel

1 Stand with your feet parallel and flat on the floor, shoulder-width apart, your knees soft, shoulders relaxed, mind clear, and breathing slowly and evenly. Let your arms hang naturally down by your sides. If necessary, or if you wish, this exercise can be performed in a sitting position, in which case it is preferable to sit upright on the edge of a chair. Do not slump, as this tends to inhibit or block the Chi.

2 Slowly raise your arms out to the sides, bringing them upward until they are directly above your head. Keep your elbows slightly bent, inhaling as your arms come up. Flex your wrists so that the flat palms are facing toward the sky. Exhale slowly.

3 As you breath in again, draw in the fresh Chi of the heavens to gather in your palms. Let your palms fill with this fresh, clean energy, as if they were sponges soaking up heavenly Chi. Feel it accumulate. When you breath out, do not let any of the Chi disperse, but hold the energy in your palms using your mind and will. Let your feet be flat and grounded on the Earth. In this position you are standing between Heaven and Earth. The energy in your palms can be directed outside of you, like the beam of a flashlight. In this exercise you will use this energy beam through the way that you angle and point your palms, and use your mind, to clean out any negative energy.

4 Slowly turn your palms over so that they are facing downwards towards the top of your head. Angle your palms so that their energy beams are directed to the point on the very top of your crown. This is the Paihui point, One Hundred Meetings, and it is one of the major Chi Kung points. Using your mind and will, send the energy that you have gathered in your palms to this point.

5 Hold this position for a moment. Feel the Chi. As you *slowly* exhale through your mouth, bring your hands and palms down in front of your body, so that your palms are facing toward the floor and the tips of the fingers of each hand are facing each other, 3–6 inches apart, as if they were resting on top of a balloon, slowly pushing it down in front of you. See them sweeping down your Conception channel (see page 57), from the top of your head all the way down to the perineum (the lowest point of your torso between your legs). Then, having reached the lowest point, let your hands go so that they are hanging naturally by your sides, and continue on down the front of your legs through and out of the soles of your feet, just by using your mind.

6 When you reach the soles of your feet, continue on down with your mind, so that you push any negative Chi out, three feet beneath you, outside of your personal energy field. Although this procedure may seem long and complex at first, after a little practice it will become easy to do it during one slow exhalation. (Do not worry if you are in a building where there are other floors and people below you. Once the negative Chi is outside your own individual field it will disperse harmlessly into the atmosphere, like a drop of liquid in an ocean.)

7 Repeat this procedure at least twice more, for a minimum of three times.

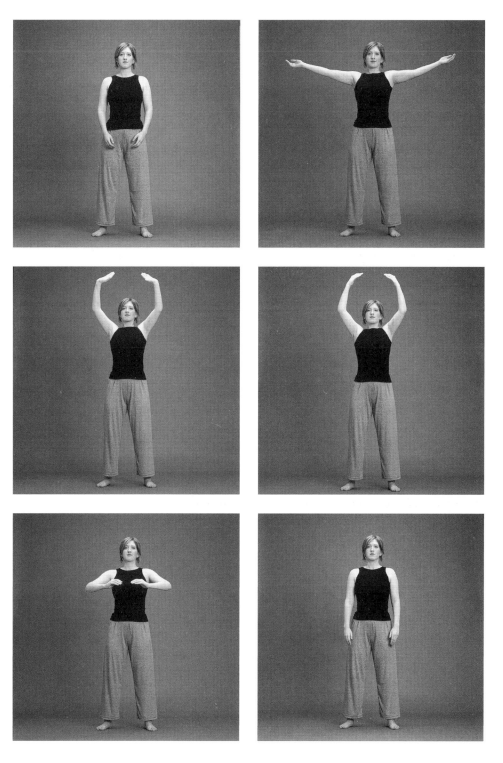

8   Repeat 1, 2, 3, and 4 above. These are the preparatory movements and you finish with your palms above your head, loaded with heavenly Chi and radiating down to your crown.

9   Hold this position for a moment. Now, as you *slowly* exhale, bring your hands and palms down facing toward the floor, but this time down your sides with your fingers pointing forward. Imagine that you are pushing down a bigger balloon than before. See the energy in your palms sweeping down through the central core of your body, in the middle of your body in front of the spine, from the top of your head to your perineum (along the Thrusting channel, *see* page 59). See the energy in your palms dragging out and cleaning any negative Chi from your central core. When you have reached the bottom of your torso and your hands are hanging by your sides, continue on down using your mind alone through the central core of your legs, to come out through the soles of your feet.

10   After reaching the soles of your feet continue on down with your mind, until you have pushed any negative Chi out three feet beneath you, outside of your energy field. Let your hands, body, and mind relax.

11   Repeat this procedure at least two more times.

Clearing the Back Channel

12   Repeat 1, 2, 3, and 4 above. These preparatory movements again end with your palms above your head, loaded with clean, fresh, heavenly Chi and radiating down to your crown.

13   Hold this position for a moment and "feel" it. Let it soak in to you. Breathe in and out slowly and savor the sensation.

14   *Slowly* breath out, and as you do let your hands descend again, with your palms facing down toward the floor, but this time with your shoulders as wide, back, and open as possible. As you bring your hands down they are now either side of your head and body, but this time with the tips of your fingers pointing toward each other. Your hands sweep down the sides of your body. As you do this, angle your palms and use your mind to direct the energy beam down the channel on the back of your head and then down the center of your back (along the Governor channel, *see* page 56). Slowly bring your palms down as if you are sweeping and cleaning any negative Chi out of the channel along the midline of your back. Run this down the central back line to the perineum, then using your mind continue on down the back of the legs and through and out of the soles of your feet.

15   When you reach the soles of your feet, again continue on down with your mind, pushing any negative Chi three feet beneath you, out beyond your energy field.

16   Let your hands, arms, body, and mind relax. Take some moments to savor the sensation and feeling.

17   Repeat this procedure at least twice more.

At the end of the whole sequence, which can be performed quickly or slowly, depending on the time that you have available and the amount of attention that you want to give to it, you will have cleaned some of the negative Chi out of your system. This is a wonderful thing to do. For the sake of the minimal effort involved in learning this simple and straightforward sequence, you can learn a skill that you can use for the rest of your life.

Do this exercise every morning to start your day. Do it at night to relax, unwind, and prepare to sleep. Do it any time you want. This practice is like taking a shower—you end up clean, fresh, and relaxed.

Focusing at your Body-Energy Center

This is an internal Nei Dan practice to increase the volume of your energy, to "ground" you, to keep you "centered" by bringing energy to your physical center, and to give you a way to "check in" with yourself.

You are going to create a "Pa Kua"—a pattern of three concentric octagons, one inside the other—around your navel. To learn how to create this pattern, and to train your mind, you should begin by using a finger to draw imaginary lines on your abdomen around your navel. Then, after you have practiced, you will be able to create it just by using your mind alone.

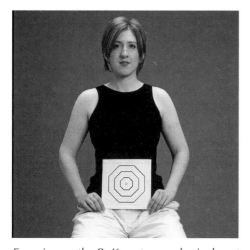

Focusing on the Pa Kua at your physical centre

Forming a Pa Kua at your Navel

1 Sit on the edge of a chair, with your knees parallel, shoulder-width apart, and bent at right angles, feet flat on the floor. This exercise can also be done lying down. Place your right hand facing down, over your left hand facing upward, and let your clasped hands rest gently in your lap. Clear your mind of extraneous thoughts and visualize a blue cloudless sky.

2 Looking down at your navel, imagine it is a clock face, with the navel as the center— twelve o'clock at the top, three o'clock to the left-hand side, six o'clock at the bottom, and nine o'clock on the right-hand side.

3 Do this exercise with your eyes half-closed—half outward-focused watching what you are doing, half inward-focused feeling the sensations that you are experiencing. Later, when you are familiar with the procedure, do it with your eyes fully closed, so that you can concentrate on the sensation and experience. In this way you will train yourself how to control and direct your energy with your mind alone.

4 Place a finger on your abdomen 3 inches above your navel at twelve o'clock. All of the lines on this octagon, 3 inches from your navel, are about $2\frac{1}{2}$ inches long. To get to the starting point on this top line, come back to your right-hand side $1\frac{1}{4}$ inches.

5 With the tip of your finger go from right to left and draw a horizontal line across the top.

6 Moving in a clockwise direction draw another line diagonally downward.

7 Next, draw a line vertically down from top to bottom on the left side, at the three o'clock position.

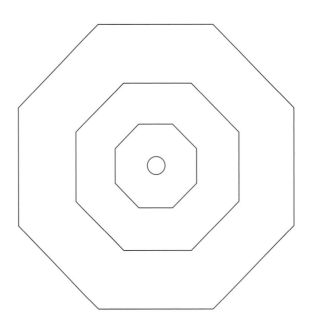

8   Then, angle diagonally inward and down.

9   Next, draw a line horizontally across the bottom from left to right at the six o'clock position.

10 Then, angle diagonally up toward the right.

11 Draw vertically up, from bottom to top, at the nine o'clock position.

12 Finally, angle diagonally inward and upward, to join the right-hand side starting position of the original horizontal line across the top.

You have now completed the first and outermost octagon of the Pa Kua.

13 Repeat the above sequence, only this time just 2 inches from the navel. Each line is approximately 1½ inches long.

14 Then, repeat the sequence, but this time only 1 inch from the navel. Each line is approximately ¾ inch long.

You have now completed all three octagons of the Pa Kua. Now do the sequence again, but without using your fingers.

15 Again draw three concentric octagons of 3 inches, 2 inches, and 1 inch, *but this time just with your mind.* Close your eyes and concentrate. Repeat this over and over again until you can feel and sense it clearly. In this way you will educate and train your mind to draw the Pa Kua, and thereby train your mind to direct and control your Chi.

16 Repeat this until you can do it at will. If you lose the sense of it, then go back to doing it with your finger. For a more direct experience, try doing it directly on your skin, not through clothing. Repeat until you "get it." By performing this procedure you form a net or web around your navel, which can collect energy there. Pa Kuas are wonderful energy collection patterns. You can also use Pa Kuas at any other points to concentrate your energy there.

Now you need to learn how to activate and "open" your energy, to "turn it on."

17 Using the tip of a finger, start in the center of your navel and begin to spiral outward, keeping your finger flat against your skin, in ever-increasing and expanding spirals (see diagrams on page 98). Men should go in a counter-clockwise direction, from twelve o'clock to nine to six to three and back to twelve. Women should go in a clockwise direction from twelve o'clock to three to six to nine back to twelve again. Move from the center all the way out to the edge of the base of the ribs at twelve o'clock, and the top of the pubic bone at six o'clock. Do nine spirals out and then reverse the direction for six spirals in. Maintain the visual image of the Pa Kua energy net while doing this. Spiraling in this direction opens the energy center and activates it.

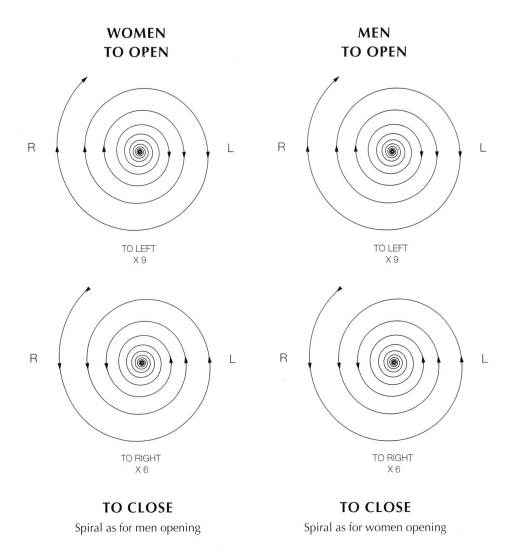

**WOMEN
TO OPEN**

R   L

TO LEFT
X 9

R   L

TO RIGHT
X 6

TO CLOSE

Spiral as for men opening

**MEN
TO OPEN**

R   L

TO LEFT
X 9

R   L

TO RIGHT
X 6

TO CLOSE

Spiral as for women opening

Opening and Closing your Body's Energy Center

18   Finally, to close your energy center, put one palm over your navel, with the center of the other palm on top of it: left hand first for men, right hand first for women. Concentrate you mind on the navel point, and imagine that you are breathing into it. It is *most* important to close down the energy center after you have finished so, after you have opened this energy center up, you *must* reverse the direction and sequence in order to safely bring your energy back to your center—to the right for women and to the left for men—otherwise it will remain opened up and may be uncontrolled.

This whole procedure brings the energy into the navel, the primary energy center and storehouse. This is where the pre-natal Chi first entered into you, as an embryo in the womb. It is Home Base. If you concentrate your energy there it will be stable and safe.

You can also use the focusing procedure to build up your energy and increase its volume. Use it whenever you need to. Use it before going to sleep. Put it on automatic and have it happen all the time, by itself. Forming and activating the Pa Kua around your navel is one of the primary techniques to control, increase, and recharge your own energy.

Advanced Practice

- Once you have mastered the procedure with just your mind, you can use it to "check in" to yourself. If this practice is difficult to do because your energy feels too wild and out of control, or because it is too sluggish and will not move easily, then this is feedback about how your energy is doing. By concentrating and establishing control over the Pa Kua you can thereby establish control of your whole energy.
- To take this procedure further and concentrate your energy even more strongly, condense your Pa Kua into 1½ inches diameter.
- To develop even more concentration and power, spiral out 36 times and in 24 times.
- To gather more energy into you, use your mind to draw external Chi from the sunlight, grass, trees and flowers, Moon, stars, heavens, and cosmos into yourself.

The Microcosmic Orbit:
Small Heaven Meditation

When we rest in the fetal position it provides us with a sense of comfort, security, protection, relaxation, and peace. The ancient Chi Kung masters discovered that the means to regain the pre-natal state of completeness lies within ourselves. You can recreate this state of perfect Chi flow in your own body through methods found in the Microcosmic Orbit/Small Heaven meditation—using movement, breath, concentration, and visualization.

The Microcosmic Orbit was developed to unify the state of harmony and balance originally experienced within the womb. Before your birth, the energy channels flowing in the front (Conception channel) and the back (Governor channel) were fully connected for a smooth flow of Chi during your pre-natal life. At birth, your flow is less completely connected, and the mouth and anus, which were previously closed, open to receive food and eliminate waste products from the body. These changes create a diminished flow and circulation of Chi within the orbit.

To accommodate these changes and help regain a state that is reflective of the peace and perfect state of pre-natal existence, Chi Kung masters developed the Microcosmic Orbit

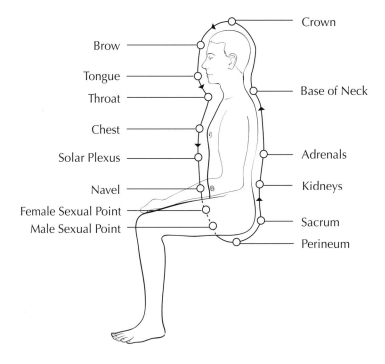

The Microcosmic Orbit

meditation to enable us to rediscover this harmony and balance by purifying the orbit of old, stagnant Chi, and by bringing fresh Chi into the body.

Preparation

1   The Small Heaven meditation can be practiced either standing or sitting. If standing, relax with your knees slightly bent, your feet shoulder-width apart, and your arms hanging with the hands and fingers very relaxed. If sitting, sit on the edge of a chair or with your back against the chair if that is more comfortable, your hands on your thighs with your palms up. Keep your feet parallel with each other, your chin parallel to the ground, and your eyes looking forward.

2   Close your eyes and allow your tongue to roll up to the palate. Then bring the tip of the tongue to the roof of the mouth toward the front teeth so that the tongue is just touching the teeth, and then just draw the tongue back a little way. You will feel where the tongue drops in. You want to rest your tongue on that ridge.

3   Sit relaxed for a few minutes, taking some deep breaths in and out, allowing the tension of the day to be released and your body to be physically relaxed. Remember, when taking a breath in you are bringing in good, clean Chi and when breathing out you are releasing all the old, stagnant Chi.

4   Now, connect all that is above with all that is below, and all that is below with all that is above, in order for their unification to occur. Remember that at each point as you

focus your attention going through the orbit, you can visualize the unified fields of those energies coming to you consciously, calling upon the direct energies of Earth and Heaven, and bringing their positive influences into your daily life and your own unique personal energy. You may picture these sources as unified in a ball of light that you hold with your mind in front of each point as you move through the orbit. Bring the energy of that ball of light into each of the points—to infiltrate and strengthen the orbit.

Practice

- **Lower Tan T'ien.** Draw your attention, and the focus of your mind and energy, to the lower Tan T'ien. Focus at the Tan T'ien and draw the energies of Heaven and Earth to you.
- **Pubic.** Draw your attention going straight down the center of the body to the pubic area, pausing at the point of the pubic bone, once again to draw the energies in and feel the depth of the movement of the orbit from within.
- **Perineum.** Now draw the energy down to the perineum calling all the energies once again into that point to merge with your own orbit energies cycling through the body.
- **Sacrum.** From the perineum the energy moves into the tailbone and from there moves straight up the lower back into the sacrum, bathing the bones with Chi and moving up to the lower lumbar region.
- **Lumbar.** Allow the energy to rise slowly through the lumbar vertebrae, one by one, from the 5th to the 1st in the region of the kidney area.
- **Thoracic.** Allow the energy to continue slowly to rise up through the thoracic vertebrae, one by one, from the 12th to the 1st, connecting at the base of the neck.
- **Cervical to Paihui.** Continue slowly up through the cervical vertebrae, one by one, from the 7th to the 1st, and bring the energy up to the occipital region, to the Paihui point at the center of the occipital bone connecting with the deep recesses of the brain.
- **Brow.** From there, moving the energy through the top of the head toward the forehead/brow, feel again the depths of the energy as it moves through the entire channel from the Tan T'ien.
- **Conception to Navel.** Next, bring the energy down from the forehead region through the tongue and the center of the face to the throat, and from the throat region, move the energy down to the center of the chest. Returning once again to the Tan T'ien level, allow the energy to build and concentrate.
- **Navel.** Allow the energy to rest at the Tan T'ien and gather there, continue collecting through the Heaven and Earth, gathering the Chi into your body, gathering it into the orbit channels. As the energy moves through your body it is being refined and applied to your own unique system. It is also being purified. It purifies you and then it is being stored.
- **Hands over Navel/Tan T'ien.** For men, slowly put your left hand over the Tan T'ien with the palm facing the body, then the right hand on top of it. For women, slowly put

your right hand over the Tan T'ien with the palm facing the body, then the left hand on top of it. Breathe in and continue to visualize gathering energy into the Tan T'ien. Breathe all the Chi into your body through the Tan T'ien.

- **Return**. When you are comfortable, begin to open your eyes and adjust back to the room. Draw your attention to how you now feel in comparison to how you felt when you began. Notice how your mind and body feel. Remind yourself to be in this energy all the time, to live with the flow of Chi.

The Macrocosmic Orbit:
Big Heaven Meditation

The Macrocosmic Orbit/Big Heaven meditation is designed to open all of the Acupuncture channels in the human body. This is a practical exercise that uses the mind to move the Chi throughout the energy pathways of the trunk, arms, and legs. When performed regularly over a period of time, a feeling as if the body is much lighter may occur.

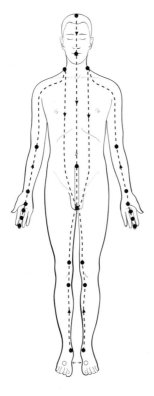
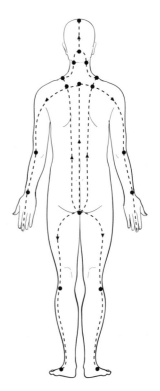

The Macrocosmic Orbit

Preparation

A prerequisite is that you have already mastered the Microcosmic Orbit/Small Heaven meditation (*see* pages 100–101). As before, this energy exercise can be performed in a sitting or lying down position. You must first make three adjustments.

- First adjustment. The body is relaxed and comfortable.
- Second adjustment. The breathing is comfortable. Slow, long, thin, soft, and even breaths will help the body relax and further the efforts of the first adjustment.
- Third adjustment. The mind must be able to concentrate in a relaxed manner. A distracted mind is unable to direct Chi. A relaxed, concentrated mind can catch the feeling of Chi and direct it to any place within the body.
- Connect the tip of the tongue to the roof of the mouth.

Practice

Circulation of the Chi Energy through the Big Heaven

1 Begin the practice by concentrating on the lower Tan T'ien below the navel. When the feeling of the Chi begins to circulate out from the Tan T'ien, the mind can then direct the Chi with the breath throughout the body.
2 Breathe out. Move the Chi to the perineum.
3 Breathe in. Move the Chi up the Governor channel, along the center of the back to the top of the head.
4 Breathe out. Move the Chi down the Conception channel, along the center of the front back down to the perineum.
5 Breathe in. Move the Chi up the sides of the back of the trunk (as if following the lines of suspenders/braces) to the area of the shoulder.
6 Breathe out. Move the Chi down the outside arms to the fingertips of both arms.
7 Breathe in. Move the Chi energy from the fingers up the inside of the arms, through the armpit area to the top of the shoulders.
8 Breathe out. Move the Chi down the front of the trunk (as if following the lines of suspenders/braces) and converge back down to the perineum.
9 Breathe in. Move the Chi inside the body through the Thrusting channel to the lower Tan T'ien. Do not go any higher than the lower Tan T'ien.
10 Breathe out. Send the Chi back down the inside of the body, splitting the Chi at the perineum. Continue, sending the Chi down the outside of both of the legs to the toes.
11 Breathe in. Move the Chi up the inside of the legs back to the perineum and inside the body to the lower Tan T'ien.
12 Breathe out. Move the chi back down to the perineum.
13 This completes one cycle of the Big Heaven Circulation. Repeat for a minimum of 9 cycles or for as long as desired. Finish the practice by rubbing the lower Tan T'ien to settle the Chi there, and end by gently rubbing the surface of your body.

Points to remember

- Always perform the three adjustments.
- Wait for the *feeling* of Chi to appear before attempting to move the Chi. If you are unable to feel the Chi, use the mind to think of the area.
- Use breath and mind together.
- Remain calm and patient, never force the Chi. Remember, the Chi follows the mind; the mind leads the Chi.
- Enjoy the feeling of nothingness as the Chi circulates in the body.
- Always finish the practice by rubbing the lower Tan T'ien to settle the Chi.

Lying, Sitting, Standing, and Moving

We usually rest when lying or sitting and use energy when standing or moving. But we can also bring resting into standing and moving, and recharge and feel comfortable while standing still. With correct practice, standing will come to feel like sitting, sitting will come to feel as restful as lying, and we can find the center point of stillness when moving.

Even the simplest lying position can be uncomfortable if your energy is out of balance or not flowing freely. Likewise, simply sitting with good posture can become difficult after a while. The same goes for standing and moving. When your energy flows freely you can remain in one position for a long period of time, resting and building energy.

When your energy "activates" and "charges up," it can move your body into exactly the correct position within moments. This will get better each time if you practice regularly, and your body will begin to remain in this energy state by itself without your even noticing it, because it is natural to assume these postures when your energy is full and flowing. It becomes much more natural than slumping, slouching, or leaning.

LYING CHI KUNG

Lying Chi Kung is mostly practiced unconsciously, while asleep. It is a form of Natural Chi Kung and we do it every night, releasing our tensions and recharging with energy for the following day. In fact, the actual recharge process can take place in a surprisingly short time. Most of us awaken a little earlier in the morning than usual and decided to go back to sleep, but then noticed that when relaxing again a gentle surge of wakefulness and energy flows into us, such that, instead of falling asleep, we wake up more. People who have experienced this often find it annoying, but it is a very precious point of mental balance and it is valuable to recognize, learn how to use, and sustain it (*see* page 167).

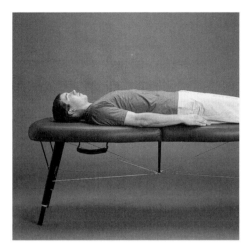

Focusing your Chi whilst lying

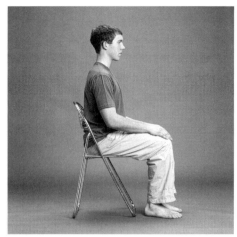

Focusing your Chi whilst sitting

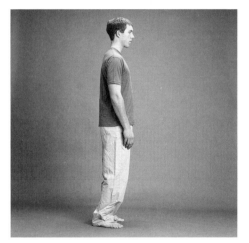

Focusing your Chi whilst standing

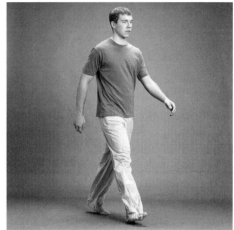

Focusing your Chi whilst moving

This is an example of how vital energy is able to flow into you when the mind relaxes in just the right way, usually at a point during sleep. Then, if your meridians are open, the energy nourishes your whole being through and through, right down to your deepest level. If you can reproduce this when sitting, standing, or even moving, you will have discovered and accomplished something within yourself of great value and benefit. You can also practice the Three Tan T'ien practices while lying (*see* page 83).

Sitting Chi Kung can be more resting and relaxing than lying down to sleep, especially when you align the three Tan T'ien well enough so that the energy flows by itself. Focus on developing the alignment of the three Tan T'ien "in a row," and learn to relax in that place, also bringing in an alignment of your mental and emotional "postures" or "balance points." The energetic occurrences during Sitting Chi Kung resemble very closely the recharge period of sleep, but the person remains awake and aware the whole time. At first the mind is used to check one's alignment with gravity, and to check energy connections within the body, such as by opening the Eight Extraordinary meridians. The mind then takes a break and observes the whole body and energy system from a viewpoint that is increasingly more tranquil and profound as you find your center.

Movement and stillness coexist within each posture. You may appear to be sitting still on the outside, but the mind and emotions may be moving about on the inside. Eventually this inner movement of the mind, emotions, and energy slows down naturally and comes to a standstill. This produces a profoundly comfortable and tranquil state of heightened awareness. During the Chi Kung State, you are cleansed, nourished, and healed to the deepest core of your being. The longer you stay there the better, and it is best to return daily. Once you experience this state, however briefly, you will want to return to enjoy it more, even if it takes a little work to get there.

STANDING CHI KUNG

Standing Chi Kung retains the spinal and Three Tan T'ien alignments learned during sitting, as well as the energy flows in the body, but while you are standing on your feet. Also, you strive to retain the actual feel of sitting while standing. When this feeling is achieved it is like sitting back on a chair, but while still standing. In this way you can rest and charge up with energy while just standing there, rather than expending energy to stand.

After you use your mind to get the energy to flow, you will need to learn to let it move through your system by keeping your mind out of the way. Using the mind to get the energy to move, as you need to do in the early stages of practice, expends mind-energy and can wear you out. Spinal and Three Tan T'ien alignment, and relaxation, are of central importance in Standing Chi Kung. It is just like balancing a pole on your hand—when the point of balance is found it takes little or no effort to keep it there, but until this point is found you will be making wild swinging movements in an effort to balance it. When the new balance is found, the pole, or your central axis, comes to rest and stillness ensues. Then, as long as you remain aware and present, it requires only minimal adjustments to remain relaxed in the aligned, balanced posture.

Standing practice is simple to get started. You can easily feel some balance, alignment, and relaxation right in the beginning, but probably only for a few seconds or a minute. So, start with one minute of practice. Be very correct, even if the practice is short, but practice frequently. Learning to stand still with correct alignment is a long-term project that leads to some of the deepest and most profound levels of Chi Kung. When your structural alignment is correct, or close enough to correct for beginners, look for that "this is easy" feeling and stay there, relaxing and doing your mindwork energy practices. Gradually, prolong your mindwork so that you are in the realm of "this is not so easy anymore," then stay there a little while to see what your body teaches you, finishing your practice before you overdo it. As with all the other Chi Kung practices, when you finish gather the Chi into your lower Tan T'ien.

MOVING CHI KUNG

Moving Chi Kung forms are done on the basis of the feelings and experiences learned in standing practice. Moving Chi Kung retains the feeling of Standing Chi Kung (which feels like sitting), while moving the arms and legs. The widely varied and diverse forms of Moving Chi Kung use hand and mind movements, to stir, refine, transform, gather, store, or discharge various kinds and levels of energy. The hand movements may brush along energy pathways, or circle around energy centers, or just hold energy in one place.

When we move, we consciously direct the body in a particular way for a specific end or purpose. This may be to achieve an external goal or to perform the movement for its own sake or just for fun. We can also move in a way that develops our energy. Chi Kung practices, and such forms and sequences as Tai Chi, are designed to develop our energy system. The more advanced the movements are, the more difficult they are to learn, but generally they lead back to the correct simplicity for a better result. It is all in these correct but simple basics—sitting and standing, then moving or lying down, without ever leaving your center.

Continuing Life Practice

Lying, sitting, standing, and moving are the most basic ways in which we inhabit and hold our bodies. Within each of these positions are countless variations. All of them can be performed without ever leaving your center, once you have trained and found it by using tranquil sitting and standing practices.

There are two central aspects to Chi Kung—Formal Practice and Life Practice. Formal Practice is the time invested in practicing particular specific exercises to develop and promote certain parts or aspects of yourself and your energy system. Life Practice is how you carry what you have developed throughout your life from moment to moment. Many people stop practicing when they end a Formal Practice sequence, but the normal activities of lying, sitting, standing, and moving are the times when you can apply and integrate what you have learned. You can practice Chi Kung lying in bed, sitting at your desk, standing in a line, or simply walking. In this way Chi Kung can become an intrinsic part of your normal daily life.

PART FOUR

More
Chi,
More
Life

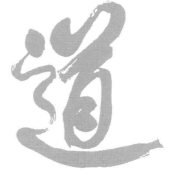

CHAPTER EIGHT

Advanced Practices

气功

The following practices are more advanced. They are modifications of high-level practices, which have been specially adapted for this book, and each one stands on its own. As an essential foundation, it is first necessary to learn the beginning practices in the previous chapter.

Do these advanced practices lightly and gently at first, until you can practice them without reference to the book, then adjust the focus and intensity, and the time spent on them to your own comfort threshold. Try them in different ways. Be creative. If you have any unexpected responses to the practices, return your energy to your navel, and seal it there safe and sound. These practices were held in secrecy for millennia in China and the East, where they were only taught to initiates, and it is only recently that they have become known in the West. They are presented here in a simplified form to give you a further sense of your energy potential. Try them and you will experience your energy in new and dynamic ways.

The Eight Extraordinary Meridians

This is an internal, Nei Dan practice that may be done at different levels of intensity. It is the basis of a nine-month training program, developed and taught by the author, that requires continued developmental practice. It is presented here in an introductory form. Try it lightly at first, and increase the intensity as you feel appropriate.

Practice

1   Sit in a comfortable position, hands on thighs in front of you. Close your eyes and focus on your breathing, clearing your mind and paying attention to your energy.

2   Focus attention at the navel and form a Pa Kua there. Open it up by spiraling in and out (see "Focusing at Your Body-Energy Center," page 95).

3   Draw external energy in to the navel as you breathe in. Accumulate energy there.

4   As you breathe out, send your Chi down to the perineum and hold it there. Feel it.

5   Breathe in and send the Chi up the Governor channel to the Paihui (One Hundred Meetings) point on the crown.

6   Breathe out and in again.

7   Connect the tip of the tongue to the roof of the mouth, on the center line at the top of the upper teeth.

8   As you breathe out, send the Chi down the front of the Conception channel to the perineum. Feel it.

9   Repeat three times, ending at the perineum.

10 As you breathe in, draw the Chi up the center line of the Thrusting channel in the middle of the body. See it as 3 inches in diameter. Slowly move it through each of the cauldrons (see Thrusting channel, page 59), and as you get to each cauldron breathe in and out again, focusing your Chi and attention there. Let it fill each cauldron. Continue up to the crown.

11 As you breathe out, move the Chi down the Thrusting channel back to the perineum, stopping at each cauldron to breathe in and out and fill each cauldron.

12 Repeat three times, ending at the crown.

13 Breathe in. As you breathe out again, descend the conception line to the navel—Home Base.

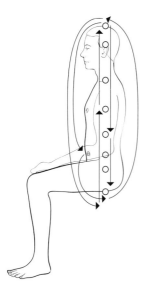

14 As you breathe in, using your mind circulate your energy around the navel to the left-hand side of the waist, around the back to the rear navel point, and then continue around to the right-hand side of the waist, back to the navel.

15 Repeat three times.

16 As you breathe in, spiral upward, turning to the left, and stopping at each horizontal point of the Microcosmic Orbit for three rotations (*see* page 89), on up to the crown.

17 Breathe in and out.

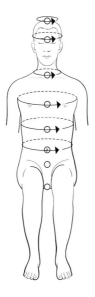

18 As you breathe out, descend, but this time rotating to the right. Stop at each point of the Microcosmic Orbit for three rotations. Continue on down to the perineum. Breathe in and out.

19 Continue on down, rotating to the right, to the knees. Rotate three times.

20 Continue on down to the soles of the feet. Rotate three times.

21 Breathe in and out.

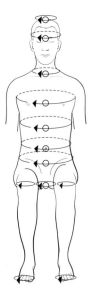

22 As you breathe in, rotate to the left three times.

23 Continue up to the knees. Rotate three times.

24 As you breathe in, continue up to the perineum.

25 Breathe in and out.

26 As you breathe, in send it up the Governor channel to the crown of the head.

27 Breathe in and out.

28 As you breathe out, send it back down the center line to the navel.

29 Hold it there.

30 Pay attention to how you now feel. Find a word, a symbol, or an image to describe how you now feel. Remember this.

31 Close down the Pa Kua by spiraling in and out (see page 98).

32 Slowly reopen your eyes and return back to the outside.

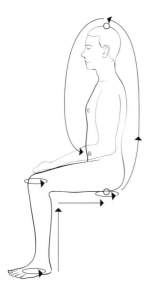

You have just opened your Eight Extraordinary meridians. Repeat this practice until you feel familiar with the sequence and the breathing patterns. The mind moves the Chi. As you become comfortable with it, try it for different numbers of breaths and at different intensities. Do not go beyond what is comfortable. If you have any adverse reactions, discontinue and try again another time. As with weightlifting, the more you practice, the stronger you get, and the more you are able to do. Take it slowly and lightly at first, then develop it further.

Advanced practice
- When you get to the Paihui point on your crown, open up the point with your mind, and draw in the external energy of Heaven as you breathe in. Add this to your Chi.
- When you get to the soles of your feet, open up the point there with your mind, and draw in the energy of Earth as you breathe in. Add this to your Chi.
- As you progress and feel familiar and comfortable, then spiral outward from the Paihui point up into Heaven, extending far out to the outer limits. Then spiral outward from your feet down to the core of the Earth.
- As you breathe in draw the energy of Heaven and Earth into you—to replenish and refresh you.
- Always bring the Chi back to your navel, and seal it there. Pay attention to how you feel. Remember it.

The Master and Coupled Points

This practice is an abbreviated form of the Eight Extraordinary meridians above, using the Master and Coupled points (*see* page 62.) It involves locating and touching these points in a specific sequence, like opening a combination lock. Because of the special function of these points they activate the Eight Extraordinary meridians in a fast and immediate way.

The names and numbers of the points are outlined in the following chart. The photographs illustrate the location of the points. When doing this practice, use your middle fingers, and focus your mind and attention to send your Chi through your fingertips into the point to turn it on. Keep your mind clear of extraneous thoughts, and pay attention to how your energy responds and feels. This practice activates the deepest core of your energy infrastructure. It is subtle and fine, so do not expect dramatic responses, but note your whole energy state afterward.

	MASTER	COUPLED
DU MO	Small Intestine 3	Bladder 62
YANG QIAO MO	Bladder 62	Small Intestine 3
REN MO	Lung 7	Kidney 6
YIN QIAO MO	Kidney 6	Lung 7
DAI MO	Gall Bladder 41	Three Heater 5
YANG WEI MO	Triple Heater 5	Gall Bladder 41
CHONG MO	Spleen 4	Pericardium 6
YIN WEI MO	Pericardium 6	Spleen 4

1 Remove any watch and bracelets, shoes and socks.
2 Begin in a sitting position, on the edge of a chair or on the floor. Concentrate on your breathing and clear your mind, focusing on your Chi.
3 With the tip of the middle finger of the right hand, touch Small Intestine 3 on the left side. Press and slightly rotate in a clockwise direction.

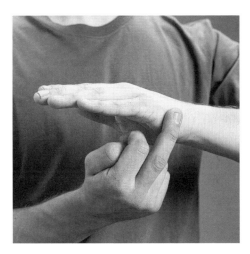

4 Now touch Bladder 62 on the left side. Press and rotate.

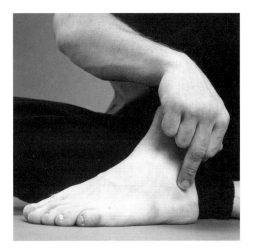

5 Now touch Bladder 62 on the right side. Press and rotate.

6 Place your hands on your knees, close your eyes, and put your attention into these four points. This activates the Governor channel and the Yang Qiao Mo. Hold your focus there. Pay attention to how this feels.

7 Open your eyes again.

8 With the tip of your right middle finger, touch Lung 7 on the left side. Press and rotate slightly in a clockwise direction.

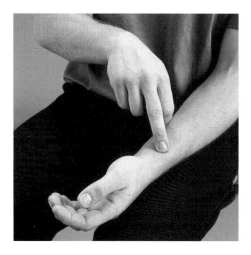

9 Now touch Kidney 6 on the left side. Press and rotate.

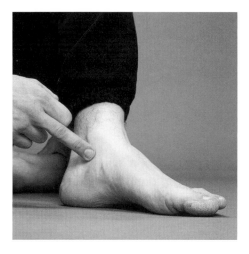

10 With the tip of the left middle finger, touch and rotate at Lung 7 on the right.

11 Repeat at Kidney 6 on the right.

12 Place your hands on your knees. Close your eyes and put your attention into these four points. Hold your focus there. This activates the Conception channel and the Yin Qiao Mo. Pay attention to how this feels.

13 Open your eyes.

14 With the tip of the middle finger of your right hand, touch Gall Bladder 41 on the left. Press and slightly rotate there in a clockwise direction.

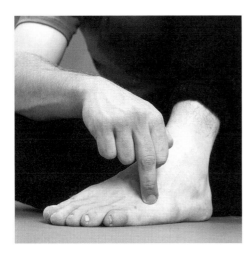

15 With the pad of the finger touch Triple Heater 5 on the left. Press and rotate.

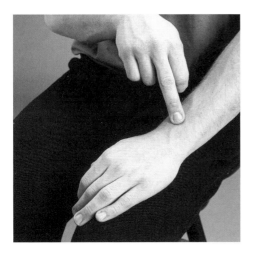

16 With the left-hand finger, touch and rotate these points on the right side.

17 Place your hands on your knees. Close your eyes and put your attention into these four points. This activates the Girdle channel and the Yang Wei Mo. Hold your focus there. Pay attention to how it feels.

18 Open your eyes.

19 With the tip of the middle finger of your right hand, touch Spleen 4 on the left side. Press and rotate slightly in a clockwise direction.

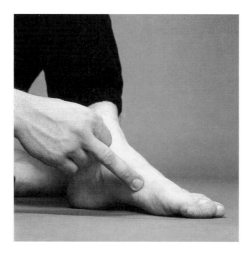

20 Touch and rotate Pericardium 6 on the left.

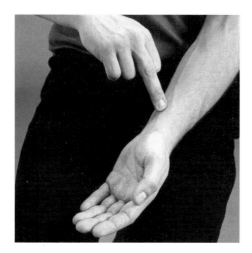

21 Reverse sides and repeat on the right side.

22 Place your hands on your knees. Close your eyes and put your attention into these four points. This activates the Thrusting channel and the Yin Wei Mo. Hold your focus there. Pay attention to how it feels. Remember this.

23 Open your eyes again.

24 Now repeat this whole sequence in one continuous sequence—left then right on each pair of channels.

25 Place your hands on your thighs. Close your eyes. Put your attention into all of these 16 points at the same time. Hold your focus. Pay attention to how your energy feels and what it does. Feel it. Experience it. Remember it.

This simple practice has activated all your Eight Extraordinary meridians. They are the foundation and infrastructure of your whole energy system.

• You can do this at any time—to revitalize and refresh you.
• With practice, the routine can be done in five minutes for an instant recharge.
• You can eventually do this with your mind alone.
• With enough practice, your energy begins to do this routine automatically and you begin to operate in your everyday at a higher level.

The External Energy Field (Wei Chi)

The body's energy system does not stop at the skin surface, but extends out around the body as an electromagnetic aura—like a pattern of iron filings extending round a simple bar magnet (see diagram on page 122). This is the Wei Chi, the External Energy Field, and it is this that connects us with the energy outside us in other people and the environment. The following is a practice to feel and experience your own field, and to draw in the energy of Heaven and Earth.

Practice

1 Breathing gently in and out through the nose, begin to think about the energy of the Earth. Visualize a place that conjures up an image of your connection with the Earth and with the ground. It could be on the ocean or by the seashore, in the woods, mountains, or valleys, or in a jungle or a garden. Remember how it feels to have your feet bare and close to the ground, and the revitalizing energy that you feel through that process.

2 Now focus on Kidney 1 (Yungchuan/Bubbling Spring) on the soles of the feet, in the middle at the base of the toes. Feel this point expanding and opening up. Using your

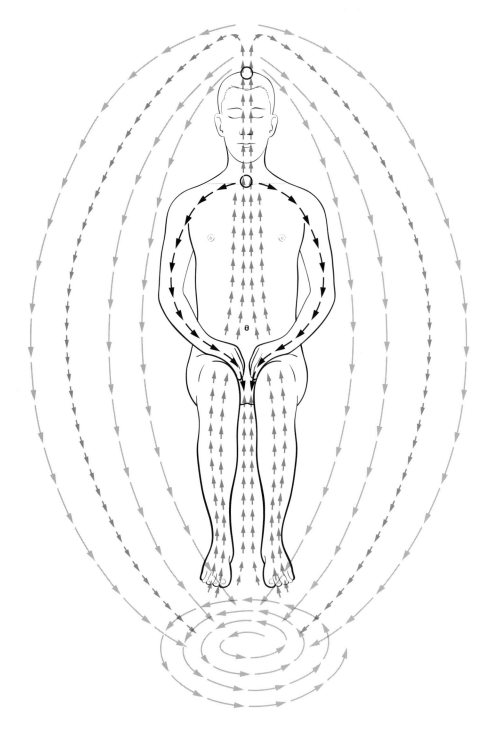

mind, imagine drawing the pure Earth energy up through the feet, into the ankles, calves, and knees. Imagine and feel the energy streaming up the center of your legs.

3   As the energy moves further up, begin to think about the body-energy that is old, fatigued, and tired; think about areas where there may be pain or disease. Feel that energy spiraling out of the body into the ground to be recycled, so that the fresh new Chi is bringing forth healing in the body as the old Chi is leaving.

4   Allow the energy to move up into the thighs and hips, and then visualize the energy moving from each of the hips into the center of the pelvis. Also, allow the area at the perineum, the beginning point for both the Governor channel and the Conception channel, to open further and to draw energy directly from the Earth into the perineum joining the two forces of energy as they come up the legs, swirling together.

5   Bring this energy straight up the inside of the middle of your body, running just in front of the spine, in your center. You can use an image that is comfortable for you, such as a pearl, a light, or a glowing flame. Feel the energy rising from the lower pelvic area, upward to the abdomen, chest, throat, base of the skull, center of the brain, and on into the top of your head. Continue to invite the pure Earth energy into your body while you expel the old. As the Chi passes through the throat area, breathe out the old Chi, expelling it down the arms and out through the hands and fingers.

6   Allow the energy to move out of the crown of your head, letting the Paihui point open, and visualize the energy now moving one or two feet above your head. Like a soft, gentle, warm rain showering down, allow the energy of the Earth to move all the way up through the body and then shower down over the whole of your body. Allow the Chi to fill the field of your aura, flowing down the front, back, and sides of you, going down past the head and neck, though the abdominal area in the front and back, filling the whole area around the pelvis. Allow the Chi to bathe the legs all the way down to the feet and allow the energy to move one or two feet underneath you, encapsulating the body from below and supporting you from below.

7   This is the energy of your own electromagnetic field. The energies of Heaven and Earth merge together, providing you with your deep connection to the origins of your life that are in the ground and the sky—your own orbit that surrounds your entire body.

The Five Animal Frolics

Over 1,800 years ago, the father of Chinese medicine, Hua To, concluded that the single greatest secret for a healthy life lay in the practice of correct movement. He created The Five Animal Frolics as a complete daily system for achieving high energy, vitality, and general well-being (*see* page 4).

The result is a delightful and accessible form of Wei Dan practice that combines an inner focus with vigorous external movement. Daily practice invigorates the internal organs and soothes the nervous system, while strengthening and toning the muscles and tendons. The Animal Frolics—as their name suggests—affirm a playful, uninhibited approach to meditative movement, generating strong benefits without being too physically demanding.

The Frolics incorporate many of the principles of Tai Chi, but in a more basic form. They are far easier to perform than Tai Chi, are very pleasurable and relatively simple to maintain as a daily practice. The student can use individual sequences as a quick, invigorating "stress-buster," or perform the full program for an exhilarating therapeutic experience.

The exercises model the movement of the Crane, Bear, Monkey, Tiger, and Deer. These are animals with very distinctive styles of movement. The idea is not merely to mimic the external motions of the animal, but to internalize the nature of that animal as you practice. Each animal corresponds to one of Chinese medicine's Five Elements, and therefore to one of the major organs. The Crane is associated with Fire and the Heart; the Bear with Water and the Kidneys; the Monkey with Metal and the Lungs; the Deer with Wood and the Liver; and the Tiger is associated with Earth and the Spleen. Therefore, each Frolic also emphasizes different health benefits, and you can choose a specific animal for specific symptoms and results.

Their movements form arcs, spirals, waves, and spins in accord with the Chinese belief that circular movement underlies all mental and subtle energetic activity. To avoid imbalance, the movements are sometimes slow, sometimes fast, and are deliberately designed alternately to strengthen or soften the body.

THE CRANE, DEER, AND STAG FROLICS

The Crane develops balance, lightness, and agility, releases the spine, and relaxes your whole body. The Deer gives a long stretch to the legs and spine, creating open, expansive movement with flexible sinews and bones. It embodies grace and relaxation.

When practicing these movements, inhale through the nose on the first movement, and exhale through the nose on the second movement. Always breathe into the lower stomach, with slow, regular, "natural" breathing. Practice at least nine repetitions of each movement. If time allows, or if you develop a special feeling or need for a particular form, do as many repetitions as you wish.

1 Place your left leg to the front, keeping all your weight on the bent right leg. Simultaneously, raise both arms out in front of your body to shoulder height, with the fingers relaxed and angled down.

2 Shift the majority of the weight onto the left leg, while opening the arms to the side of the body, shoulder height, with palms facing forward.

3 Shift the majority of the weight onto the right leg, arcing the arms down to the sides of the torso and finally just behind the torso, with palms facing back.

4 While the weight is still on the right leg, turn the left foot out at a 45° angle, then step forward with the right leg and repeat the movement to the other side.

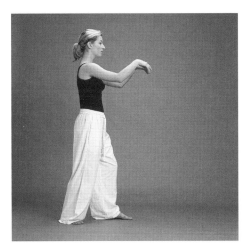
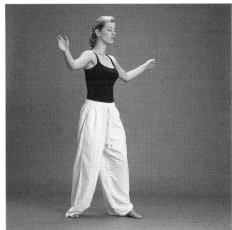
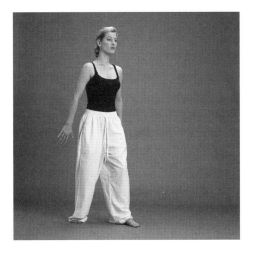

1   Step out with the left leg to the front, keeping your weight back on the bent right leg. Simultaneously, bend the waist slightly, rotate your torso to the left, move the left arm behind the body, palm up, and extend the right arm to the front, palm up.
2   Raise the left foot up to the right knee, then put it back down to its original position.
3   Step forward with the right leg and repeat the whole sequence to the other side.

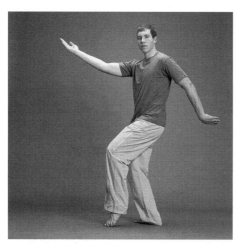 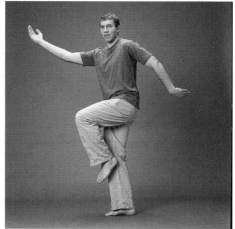

1 Begin with your heels touching and feet at a 45° angle. Bend your knees. Make relaxed fists and hold them in front of the lower stomach.

2 Step forward with the left leg, bringing both arms up simultaneously in front of the body, shoulder width, shoulder height. Have about 60 percent of the weight on the left leg. Curve the wrists slightly and relax the hands.

3 Shift more weight onto the left leg while extending the left arm and drawing the right hand along the inside of the left arm until it is opposite the left elbow. Simultaneously tilt the head to look back and up 45° to the right.

4 Continue by drawing the right hand in close to the chest. Turn the right hand to face the floor and move the palm down the front of the torso to the lower stomach.

5 Shift your weight into the right, back leg, bringing your relaxed fists to the stomach.

6 Step forward and repeat to the other side.

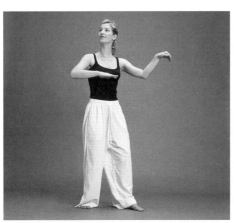
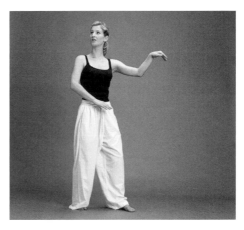
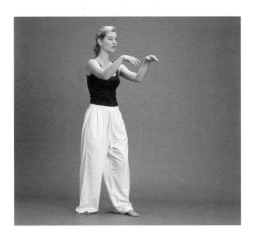
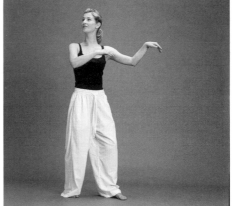

1   Begin with your heels touching and feet angled out at 45°. Bend your knees. Make relaxed fists and hold them in front of the lower stomach.

2   Raise the fists all the way up the front of the body until they are above the head, with the elbows slightly bent. Simultaneously, raise the left foot up in front of the right knee.

3   Step down, with the left instep angled out, placing the right knee into the middle of the left calf. Keep the arms up above the head. The body is turned to the left diagonal.

4   Circle the fists down to the stomach and repeat the full sequence to the right diagonal.

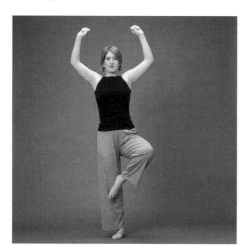 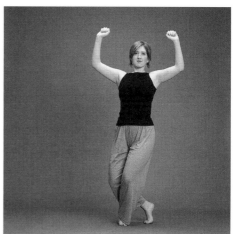

Cultivating Sexual Energy

Sexuality is a universal way for people to access quickly the flow of their Chi. The ancient Taoists developed many methods for tapping the power of sexual energy in order to direct it toward creating better physical health, a greater sense of vitality and zest for life, and to refine the sexual impulse into a steady state of spiritual bliss. Sexual Chi Kung can heal sexual dysfunction and impotence, improve sexual relationships, and relieve PMS and other menstrual difficulties.

At the core of all Chi Kung is the cosmic Yin–Yang pulsation of polarized energy around a neutral pole. Think of creation as a continuous cosmic orgasm, and the human orgasm as an exquisite echo of that pulsation. When you get these in rhythm and harmony, your personal "energy gates" open to the cosmic flow of light and love.

There are two major paths in cultivating sexual energy:

- **Single Cultivation, in which you harmonize your male–female pulsation as "internal love-making," which is only possible because every person has both Yin (female) and Yang (male) Chi within their body, regardless of their sex.**
- **Dual Cultivation, in which you exchange Yin and Yang Chi with a lover or partner.**

Sexual Chi is said to originate in the kidneys and bone marrow, and in the Chinese view this includes the penis or vagina/uterus, prostate or ovary glands, the bladder and kidney organs and their meridians, and in women also the breasts. All are part of the "water element" that regulates the body's Jing or sexual body-essence (*see* Jing Chi Shen, page 65.)

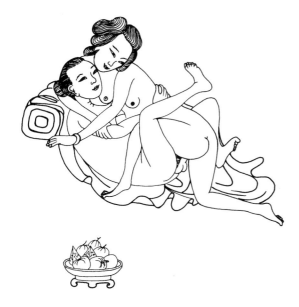

THE PROPERTIES OF SEXUAL CHI

There are two notable qualities that differentiate Sexual Chi from other kinds of Chi. Firstly, it is very "sticky," acting as the stabilizing or bonding energy between opposing Male/Yang and Female/Yin forces. Secondly, it has the power to amplify or multiply whatever it bonds to, so it intensifies emotions, multiplies cellular and glandular reproduction rates, either in one's own body or by birthing children. It can also multiply the creative energy in the worlds of work or play.

THE EXHAUSTION OR LOSS OF SEXUAL CHI

There are several ways by which precious Sexual Chi may be lost or exhausted. Some of these differ between men and women.

Men

This is typically through excessive sex and ejaculation. "Excessive" varies by body type, age, and climate, but particular care needs to be taken during the winter, when Chi is normally going in deep, not outward. There are methods of slowing down ejaculation during sex so that men can "draw out" the essence from their sperm and recycle it around the body, so nourishing other centers. It is not necessary to become celibate. These practices include "Testicle Breathing" (*see* page 132) and "Drawing Up the Golden Nectar."

The goal is to shift from a limited "genital orgasm" to a "whole body orgasm." Slowing or stopping "ejaculation" does not prevent a man from having an "orgasm" or being "multi-orgasmic." Ejaculation is physical; orgasm is your Chi pulsating. Do not get obsessed with preventing ejaculation, but focus instead on opening up your Chi channels and recycling Sexual Chi until you finally ejaculate. This also slows the man down, enabling him to stay in closer harmony with the woman's slower cycle of arousal.

Women

Excessive bleeding during the menstrual cycle causes loss of Jing. By energetically detoxifying the body with Sexual Chi Kung before the cycle begins, the need for bleeding as a means of detoxifying is vastly reduced. With a higher level of practice, the menstrual cycle can even be stopped. This practice is called "Slaying the Red Dragon." Women can also train to redirect their Sexual Chi flow up to the higher energy centers in the heart and brain.

Both sexes

Poor diet, shallow breathing, and negative emotions and mental attitudes, will exhaust your sexual vitality. Improving these, together with a regular external Chi Kung practice of at least 20 minutes daily, are the mainstay of preventing low sexual energy and the many associated dysfunctions.

It is also important to understand the relation between the Fire Element in the heart and the Water Element in the kidneys. The Fire and Water essences stimulate each other as well as keeping each other in check. It is necessary to maintain proper exchange between them, so that they attain a steady state. This can be achieved by breathing gently between the middle and lower Tan T'iens, through visualization, and by guiding Chi through the right channels. Simply by keeping an open heart you protect against blind lust, which ultimately injures the kidneys because it can never be satisfied by physical sex alone. The kidney Shen needs touch and sexual stimulation, but also it always seeks the love of the heart Shen.

Caution!

Sexual Chi is much more powerful than most people realize. We all know how long it takes people to recover from broken relationships. For this reason, it is essential that you properly prepare your energy field with Chi Kung practice for several months before attempting ovarian or seminal Kung Fu. If Sexual Chi is misdirected into the wrong energy channels, the result may range from mild discomfort to severe impairment of physical health.

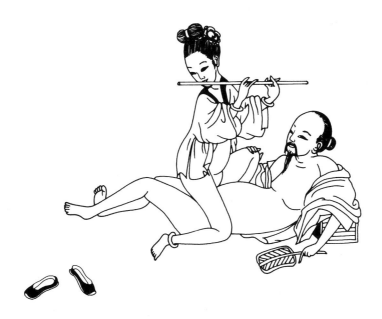

1   Learn the Five Animal Frolics and the Six Healing Sounds (see page 124) to release trapped negative emotional Chi. (There are numerous versions of these practices. They are simple, and can easily be learned from books or tapes available through magazines, book stores, and catalogs listed in the resource section at the end of this book, see pages 197–8.) They release the Chi trapped in each of the five vital organs. You do not want to amplify unconsciously old trapped feelings with supercharged Sexual Chi. Do not practice while in any extreme emotional state.

2   Practice the Healing Smile (see page 89). This insures a calm and balanced mind when you do the sexual practice.

3   Learn the Microcosmic Orbit (see page 99). This gives the Sexual Chi a safe pathway up the back and down the front of the body, with automatic "safety overflow" valves into other major meridians. If you do not learn this, there is a danger of some people getting "kundalini psychosis"—too much Chi in the brain leading to delusional states. Any Chi practice that opens the lower Tan T'ien will also prepare you and ground you.

4   Once the Microcosmic Orbit is open, it is much easier to balance the Chi flow to the endocrine glands—the adrenals, pineal and pituitary, thymus, heart and spleen, and gonads. These glands regulate the body metabolism during sexual arousal, and their healthy functioning is essential to get the benefits of the sexual practice.

It is advisable to find a teacher to help you to train. Sexual Chi Kung is not an end in itself, but merely a step within the larger process of cultivating and refining your Chi. At the same time, you should practice some form of standing Chi Kung, learning to ground the volatile Sexual Chi (see page 106).

The higher level of Sexual Chi Kung is known as "inner sexual alchemy," and through this you may become aware of the role of Shen and the vital organ spirits, in the regulation of your inner Yin–Yang balance.

Ovary and Testicle Breathing

Once you have learned the Microcosmic Orbit meditation you are ready to try other practices that utilize the same two energy channels. Ovarian and Testicle Breathing can recapture energy that is normally lost or not re-channeled. For women, Ovarian Breathing can alleviate many menstrual problems and provide a smooth transition through menopause. For men, Testicle Breathing can increase memory and clarity of mind while also reducing the desire for ejaculation. Although quite subtle to practice, these exercises can be profound in their effects.

While you are reading this, your body may be making sperm, maturing an egg, increasing the thickness of the uterine lining, or making seminal fluid—processes that we are not aware of participating in, yet they are processes that involve our most refined substances. When you embark on Chi Kung ovarian or testicular practices, your body learns to recycle your sexual energy into your reservoir of daily Chi, so that you have more creative energy to work with in your day. Your Inner Alchemy will also have a reservoir of sexual essence (Jing) ultimately to transform into spiritual energy (Shen). The transformation of Jing into Shen remains the ultimate purpose of the sexual exercises.

As you begin to conserve and transform your inner resources, you are on the road to experiencing a renewed connection between your heart and your genitals. Women feel more harmonized with their reproductive functions, and in control of their aroused sexual energy. Men become more in touch with their feelings and emotions. These changes can create greater harmony between men and women. Besides, the practice feels wonderful, sending pleasurable currents of energy up your spine to your brain.

Practice

This exercise consists of simultaneously inhaling and lifting your perineum and then, by guiding your breath up your Governor channel, drawing your sexual energy from your ovaries or testicles up to your crown, letting it spiral there for the remainder of that breath, and then exhaling, relaxing, and letting your attention come back to your navel.

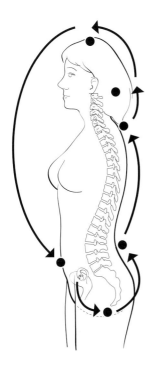

1   While sitting in a chair, with your hands lightly clasped in your lap or resting on your knees, simultaneously start to inhale a slow even breath through your nose and gently pull up your perineum. The movement of your perineum is subtle; any less would be nothing at all. When you lift up on your perineum, you are drawing energy from your ovaries or testicles to your sexual center energy point (ovary or sperm palace—*see* Microcosmic Orbit practices and illustrations). Exhale and relax.

2   Simultaneously, start to inhale a slow even breath through your nose, gently pull up on your perineum, and gently squeeze your anus. This helps bring energy from your sexual center to your perineum. Exhale and relax.

3   Again, inhale while lifting up your perineum, squeeze your anus, and now tilt the bottom of your sacrum slightly to the back of your chair. Exhale and relax. This starts your energy moving up your Governor channel.

4   Repeat this pattern, bringing energy up to your mid-back between the 11th and 12th thoracic vertebrae, the point of the adrenal glands. Exhale and relax.

5   Repeat this pattern, bringing energy up to the point between your neck and your back, Governor 14, (Tachui/Great Hammer). Exhale and relax.

6   Repeat this pattern, bringing energy up to the base of the skull, Governor 16 (Fengfu/Wind Palace). Exhale and relax.

7   Repeat this pattern, bringing energy up to your crown, Governor 20 (Paihui/One Hundred Meetings). Let your energy spiral in your crown for the remainder of your breath (do not hold your breath), and exhale, guiding your breath down your Conception channel to your navel, and relax.

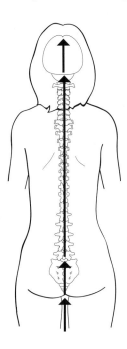

1 Sit in a chair, hands lightly clasped on your lap or resting on your knees, the tip of your tongue lightly touching your palate behind your upper front teeth.

2 Smile to your ovaries or testicles. Thank them for providing you with needed hormones and for preparing your body to reproduce. Feel gratitude for the complexity and mystery of life.

3 Simultaneously, start to inhale slowly and evenly through your nose and gently lift up your perineum. As you start to squeeze lightly your anus and tilt your sacrum, you may feel some warmth, humming, or buzzing as your sexual energy starts to move.

4 With your breath, and your inner eye, guide your energy up your Governor channel to your crown. Let your energy spiral in your crown (the direction is not important), and when you are ready to exhale, let your breath and mind flow down your front, along the Conception channel to your ovaries or testicles again. Repeat this process two more times.

5 On the third cycle, let your energy spiral in your crown and on your exhalation let your energy flow down your Conception channel to your navel. Exhale and rest for a couple of breaths.

6 Repeat this process of three breaths—the first two returning to your perineum and source of your sexual energy, and the third ending at your navel.

7 Repeat the whole sequence for 2–10 minutes, or as long as you feel comfortable. Do not overdo it at first.

8 When you have decided that you are finished, end with a few minutes of Microcosmic Orbit meditation. It is very important to do this, as it moves your energy, preventing it from getting stuck, blocked, or stagnant in your sexual centers, heart center, or brain. Finish by collecting your energy in your navel.

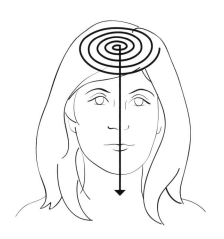

Note for women
Ovarian energy is considered warm in Chinese medical terms. It is important that this energy is not left in the brain, but instead returned to the navel every three breaths.

Note for men
Unaroused sexual energy (testicle breathing) is considered cool in Chinese medical terms. Although some instructions may say that this energy can be retained in the brain, it is always safer to bring it back to the navel.

CHAPTER NINE

Clinical Chi Kung Treatment

Clinical Chi Kung is the application of Chi Kung in a clinical context, for the treatment of illness, symptoms, and disease. There is a wide range of styles, known by such names as Chi Kung Healing, Medical Qigong, and Qigong Therapy. There are also various forms of physical manipulation treatment, and one of these, Chi Nei Tsang, is described here. No commonly agreed standards or credentials have yet been accepted in the West, since these applications are new and tend to reflect the training and viewpoint of particular schools or individuals. Discussions regarding standards, credentials, and national examinations are underway and will no doubt be agreed on by all parties in due course. What follows represents a cross-section of approaches, and the viewpoints of the respected individual contributors.

Chi Kung Healing

(*From a Classical/Pre-Communist perspective*)

Chi Kung Healing (CKH) relates to two distinct areas:

- External Chi Healing (ECH)—treatment by the healer;
- Self-Practice—self-treatment by the individual, often recommended by the healer.

CKH is a holistic integrated approach to health and healing, strong in prevention as well as treatment of illness and imbalance. Although symptoms are considered, most Chi Kung healers have a way of assessing the actual state of the energy body, and this directs the treatment process, as well as the self-practices recommended to the individual. This form of Chi Kung does not "do to" individuals as much as it "does with" them.

EXTERNAL CHI HEALING—ASSESSMENT

This is performed in many styles, often intuitively. It involves reading some or all of these aspects of the energy body:

- Wei Chi (external energy field);
- Three Tan T'ien (energy fields within, and extending out from, the body);
- Cauldrons (seven or more);
- Eight Extraordinary meridians (including the Master and Coupled points that rule them);
- Twelve major organ meridians (some of the points along these meridians, such as the source, junction, entry or exit, or Five Elements points);
- Twelve major organs (including extra organs and glands);
- Five sense organs (as windows to the outside world for the organs);
- Hara or "eye in the Solar Plexus" (and to what degree it is open);
- Any extra, aggressive, or disturbing energy in the system that needs to be dispelled;
- The balance of the Five Elements in relationship to each other;
- Stagnation (tight, not moving), excess (too much), or deficiency (too little) of Chi held in the elements/organs.

The assessment reveals an integrated picture of Body (physical), Soul (emotional), and Spirit (mental and spiritual)—always reflected in the signs and symptoms the person is experiencing, but also revealing to the trained practitioner what underlies them.

EXTERNAL CHI HEALING—TREATMENT

The treatment is carried out by using the hands and/or the mind. It stimulates the movement of energy in "blocks" revealed in the assessment. Treatment can be very specific—targeted to points, meridians, organs, or blocked areas—or more general. Usually, it is a combination of these, starting with general movement/activation of energy in the field and body (which relaxes and deepens the state of consciousness), then going on to specific treatment in the areas causing problems "down line," then again followed by general treatment to re-

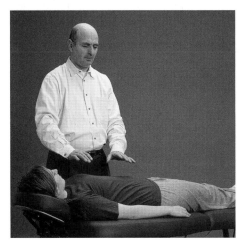

Assessing Chi

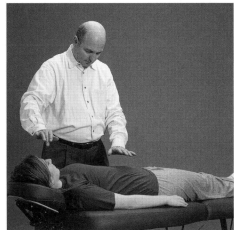

Emitting Chi

harmonize the system, ending with a grounding method. Knowing the symptoms can help, but usually the treatment and the practice recommended are related to a deeper picture of the person, understood through assessment and really "receiving" them.

PRACTICE

Chi Kung Healing always includes practice by the individual (both the person seeking help and the healer). This self-practice is considered the foundation of CKH because what you do for yourself has the most profound effects on the system and because daily practice is like daily self-treatment. Usually it is recommended to start with simple, general forms to help the system gradually start shifting toward a more balanced pattern. After this, specific practices are recommended to strengthen the constitution, temperament, or character (Jing, Chi, and Shen) through its "weakest link"—the "key" to the individual at that time.

While personal practice is the foundation of healing, most people (especially if ill or weakened) will benefit greatly from individual treatment to help name, understand, and open the most blocked areas, so that practice can proceed more smoothly. This is not always essential, but it is often desirable and helpful. The Chi Kung healer will be able to watch the progress of personal practice through the assessment of the energy-body and thus be able to help tailor the practice forms as required.

Chi Kung Healing pre-dates what has become known as Traditional Chinese Medicine (TCM), and it is usually simpler, with a strong basis in classical Taoist roots. It is almost impossible to carry out Chi Kung Healing treatment or practice on an isolated, symptom-based approach, because you are always working with the complete picture. The practitioner watches the individual's expression of energy through thought, picture, sensation, emotion, and body. These cannot be separated because they are superimposed. Most Chi Kung healers in the West use psychology as an integrated part of the healing process, because they understand the dance between:

- Jing (spirit/essence in full physical expression in the body and organs);
- Chi (the energy/vitality of essence pulsating through all the meridian streams and expressed in the emotions); and
- Shen (the consciousness/spirit of essence expressed in thoughts and pictures through the many levels of mind).

To most Chi Kung healers these are all material, but are simply much less dense than conventional physical symptoms. They can help the individual receive the "expression" of their own consciousness through their energy body (in treatment or practice) by means of body area, sensation, emotion, picture, meaning, and the need for observation or change. The healer does not usually gather this information, but instead "holds the space" for the individual to gather this understanding and thus become empowered.

CENTERING AND THE SOLAR PLEXUS BOWL

These are two Chi Kung Healing practices that have been found to be most effective. "Centering" is used to train a person's awareness to drop in to the Chi Kung State, and the "Solar Plexus Bowl" is used to re-open a major energetic door, and shift the energy-body out of stress response and into relaxation response.

These can both be done as self-practice (as described here) or as part of treatment with another person. These practices have been developed to empower people to engage more fully with their own healing process.

Centering
This practice can be done in any position, and takes about 5–10 minutes at first.

1 Bring awareness to your breath.
2 As you exhale, let your breath help you let go of any expectations.
3 As you exhale, let your breath help you let go of any effort.
4 Bring your awareness to the center of your chest (the center of your energy-body).
5 As you exhale, let your chest soften and relax.
6 Let your awareness drop in, from mid-chest (your Heart Center), as if you were slowly and gently falling or spiraling backward toward Center, an inner place of rest, between awake and asleep.

7	Allow any doors or barriers to Center to open to you.

8	Sink deeper into this inner place of rest.

9	Allow yourself to perceive the "presence" there in Center — if you are willing, surrender backward into those inner arms.

10	Resting there deep in Center, hold the question, "What is here now?"

11	Remain aware and receptive, with no expectations, no effort—at rest between your outer world and your inner world.

This is your Center Place, an internal state of consciousness, another aspect of the "Chi Kung State." From here you can proceed with Chi Kung Healing—treatment or practice. With practice you will drop into Center much faster, because your energy-body is entrained.

Solar Plexus Bowl

This practice can be performed in any position, but it is a good practice to do in bed before going to sleep at night, or getting up in the morning. It takes about 10 minutes at first.

1	Resting your mind in Center, become aware of your solar plexus — as if you were witnessing it from Center.

2	As you exhale, imagine sending your breath there.

3	Feel the area and notice the quality, sensation, or image that is there.

4	Lightly place your hands on your solar plexus with your fingertips in a straight line from your navel to the bottom of your breastbone. Your thumbs are not used except as a vent. Your fingertips are just lightly touching your body (wearing clothes is fine).

5	Image a bowl inside your solar plexus area facing up; the surface of your skin is the top of the bowl.

6	Let the energy of your fingertips sink down into the area, as if they are sinking into the bottom of the bowl.

7	Watch and feel your willingness to allow this area of your body to soften, relax, and begin to open like the eye of a camera. Feel your willingness to let go of the habit of overprotecting and unnecessarily guarding and shielding. You filter your own light out by doing that. Effort and work (pushing your fingers way in) will not help. It will only close tighter.

8	You will start to feel a physical response as your body begins to let go of your unconscious stress response and sink slowly into relaxation response.

9	Gently run your hands around the bowl's edge, pausing to let them sink to the bottom in various places, then return to the midline.

10	Imagine an egg of light all around you like a translucent shell. This is your true filter.

11	When you are ready, take in a deep breath and then, as you exhale, let your mind lead your breath down and out of your solar plexus. Keep doing this as you lift your hands off your body — drawing this old pattern of energy out. Be glad to let it go.

Each time you exhale, fill your solar plexus with breath and light, and keep drawing your hands away and out from your solar plexus bowl. You can even circle your hands out clockwise.

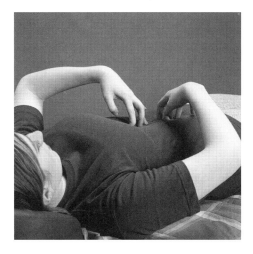 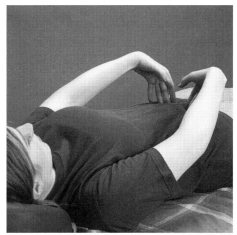

There is nothing "bad" leaving you during this practice, just an old habit of protection that has been subconsciously keeping your body in stress response, so weakening your constitution, because it was filtering your own light from full descent into your physical body. Once you have developed this process, it becomes quicker and you can do it with your mind—the mind leads the Chi.

If you do this once or twice a day, for 10 minutes each time, it will train your energy-body to respond quicker and deeper each time. This energy center will become stronger, as will your constitution (elements, organs, and meridians). Gradually, your "Solar Plexus Eye" will become more and more open until it functions at 80–100 percent all the time, instead of only up to 30 percent as with most people. Your whole life will feel and be different. This will be reflected in your body, emotions, thoughts, work, and relationships, and it will be an invaluable tool for life. Once you have tried it and felt its benefits, teach it to others.

Medical Qigong Therapy

(From the Traditional Chinese Medicine (TCM)/Post-Communist perspective)

Medical Qigong Therapy is the oldest of the four branches of Traditional Chinese Medicine and provides the energetic foundation from which Acupuncture, Herbal Healing, and Chinese Massage originated. It is through an understanding of Qigong that the other branches of Traditional Chinese Medicine are elevated to a spiritual path of self-realization and internal transformation. Doctors of Traditional Chinese Medicine address the patient's physical, energetic, and spiritual needs simultaneously. According to the principles of Traditional Chinese Medicine, the root cause of all disease can be traced to a critical imbalance within the body's vital energies. Therefore, the best way to prevent or cure disease entails establishing a healthy energetic balance and harmony between the body's energy field, and the forces of nature and the cosmos.

All of the four main branches of TCM are built on the same foundation of energetic diagnosis known as the Five Main Roots of Traditional Chinese Medicine. The Five Main Roots are used for internal organ diagnosis according to the theories of the

- Six Stages;
- Five Elements;
- Eight Principles;
- Triple Burners; and
- Four Levels.

There are many colleges of Traditional Chinese Medicine throughout China today that focus on Medical Qigong training, offering comprehensive, government-sponsored, three-year programs in Medical Qigong therapy. Programs include classes, labs, and seminars on:

- traditional Chinese medical theory;
- foundations of Chinese medicine for internal diseases—The Yellow Emperor's Inner Canon, Spiritual Axis, Essential Questions, and the Canon of Perplexities;
- energetic anatomy and physiology;
- diagnosis and symptomatology;
- energetic psychology;
- Qigong pathology;
- Medical Qigong therapy;
- Western anatomy and physiology;
- Western internal diseases;
- Health and recovery.

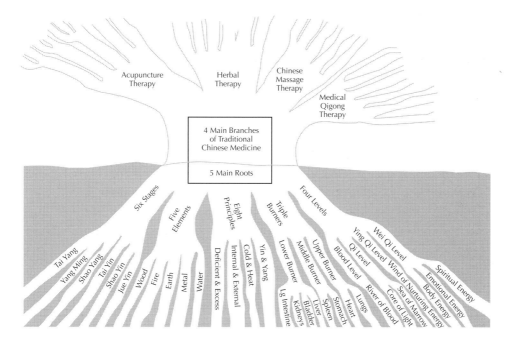

In addition, there is a survey of other related medical modalities, such as comprehensive understanding of herbal medicine, Acupuncture, and Chinese massage.

The strategy for healing disease in Medical Qigong training is threefold:

1 Eliminating internal pathological factors (the accumulation of Excessive emotions, such as anger, grief, worry, and fear), as well as external pathogenic factors (such as the invasion of Cold, Hot, and Damp from the environment).
2 Increasing or decreasing the patient's Qi as needed, to counteract the Deficient or Excessive condition within the internal organs and channels.
3 Regulating and balancing the patient's Yin and Yang energy to bring it back into harmony.

This unique therapy consists of regulating the body's three external Wei Qi fields (physical, mental/emotional, and spiritual), and four internal fields of life-force energy (Ying Qi, Sea of Blood, Sea of Marrow, and the central core Taiji Pole). Some of the most common diseases treated in Medical Qigong clinics include:

• diabetes
• arthritis
• high blood pressure
• breast and ovarian cysts and tumors

• migraine headaches
- fibromyalgia
- insomnia
- acute abdominal pain
- irritable bowel syndrome
- deep tissue obstruction
- muscle atrophy
- brain tumors
- stroke
- coma retrieval
- cancer (certain types)

Medical Qigong Therapy uses five major clinical techniques:

Distance Therapy (also called External Qi Therapy, Qi Emission, and Outgoing Qi Therapy) requires the Qigong doctor to manipulate a patient's Qi by focusing on the energetic properties of the patient's channels, collaterals, and points, as well as internal organs, from a distance of several inches, several feet, or even several miles away.

Self-Regulation Therapy (also called Qigong Prescriptions, and Patient Homework) are Qigong exercises (such as postures, movements, sound vibrations, and visualizations) given to the patient by a doctor. Patients can use these Qigong techniques to regulate their own health, using various lying, sitting, moving, and standing postures. The patient may also use their own spiritual belief systems as a healing tool.

Qigong Massage Therapy, a soft-tissue regulation technique differs from Tui Na or An Mo (Chinese External Massage Therapy), in that the doctor's hand skims the patient's body as lightly as a feather, never exceeding the pressure one would place on an eyeball. This light skimming action is used to dredge the patient's external channel Qi, causing energy to be released from the internal channels which serve as a pathway for Qi transference.

Energetic Point Therapy is used by the doctor to extend Qi into specific internal and external areas of the patient's body to lead and direct Qi. This type of therapy requires the doctor and the patient to focus their attention onto a specific energetic point. This therapy demonstrates the power of the mind as an active tool in healing, and is used for purgation, tonification, and regulation.

Invisible Needle Therapy involves the visualization of imaginary needles of light being inserted into specific points on the patient's body. The needles of light are used to stimulate and direct the patient's Qi.

Chi Kung as Therapy

(*From the Family Lineage Tradition perspective*)

Chi Kung was first applied as a field of medicine for the treatment of illness many thousands of years ago, and Chi Kung Therapy follows directly from this early tradition.

The basic therapeutic principle behind the effectiveness of Chi Kung Therapy is its ability to have a restorative value for vitality, and a storage increase capacity for energy. Chi Kung also replenishes depleted energy, the body-energy reserves that have been lost through disease or physical exertion. It encourages proper rest and recuperation, aiding our physical and mental systems toward a normal organic function. The deeply relaxing stage, achieved by the practice of Chi Kung, suppresses the excitation of the cerebral cortex. This internal inhibition engenders a calm, quiet state for extended periods, and provides for the restoration of the brain to its normal calm and alert condition. Hyperactivity is subdued by internal control, resulting in the central nervous system becoming calmer and thus more conducive to the recovery of health and vitality.

Physiological studies where Chi Kung is practiced have shown an energy-storing phase. This refers to a state where oxygen consumption is reduced by 30–35 percent, and the metabolic rate decreases around 20–25 percent. This energy boosts one's effectiveness in combating chronic and debilitative conditions, and aiding those with a weak physical constitution.

Chi Kung Therapy is a holistic approach that deals with the basic cause of disease. It also improves the function of nerve control centers, making the immune system more effective, and so aiding the self-cure from a number of diseases at the same time. The Chi Kung state is one where the thinking mind is at rest and the body is totally calm and relaxed. For instance, increased perspiration can be brought about by vasodilation in the extremities and by increasing peripheral circulation, both of which can improve the complexion. The skin can become softer and smoother. Also, there is an increase in metabolic process, improving the distribution of nutrients from food and blood throughout the system. A feeling of expansion, increased warmth, and an overall sense of well-being can result.

Chi Kung can correct conditions such as digestive disorders, respiratory problems, nervous dysfunction, and reproductive ailments. It can also aid recovery after major surgery, and help in recuperation and convalescence.

To obtain maximum benefits for people who are very ill, the practice of Chi Kung should be undertaken with a complete break from having to attend to the details, responsibilities, and cares of everyday life. The individual concerned will need an area of quiet, care, and support. If Chi Kung is practiced in an environment that encourages concentration, peace, and harmony, this will increase and conserve vital energy, as well as providing the surplus energy necessary to activate the powerful internal mechanisms and assure that one's inner resources are quickly restored. In this way Chi Kung improves the constitution, builds health, and prevents disease.

Chi Nei Tsang (Internal Organ Chi Massage)

Chi Nei Tsang translates as "Energy–Internal–Yin-Organs." It is one of a wide range of techniques which use physical manipulation as well as energy, and it is presented here as an example of other ways of working in clinical treatment. It is a series of exercises and practices to develop a deeper understanding of bodywork and its relation to Chi. These techniques use visceral manipulation and energy work to open up energy in the lower Tan T'ien and redistribute the life force through the organs and meridian system. In time, a transformation occurs and many illnesses can be helped and optimal health obtained.

Chi Nei Tsang (CNT) is a Taoist system of healing massage that focuses on the navel center of the body. It is thought that the navel center is the primary area where imbalances occur that may cause negative emotions, stress, tension, congestion, and illness. Using visceral manipulation and energy work, CNT techniques provide a method to balance the energy, thereby improving many vital body functions. Practitioners use a variety of light and deep manipulation techniques to help restore function within the internal organs, connective tissue, tendons, muscles, lymph, nerve, and endocrine system. It is part of a larger Taoist paradigm of practice that includes meditation, Tai Chi, and Chi Kung. CNT techniques are easily adaptable for self-practice, thereby offering the individual the opportunity to both heal themselves and learn practices so that they can take better care of themselves.

CNT incorporates the Taoist understanding of the meridian systems and the cultivation of energy to keep healthy and create vitality. These precise techniques enable energy blockages to be cleared in the abdominal area and within the internal organs long before it is noticed in the periphery of the body.

Some of these techniques only work with the body's extremities and energy channels, far from the navel center and the organs. Chi Nei Tsang has been called a most "direct system," working with the Tan T'ien, a source for all meridians and energy channels.

Sessions are carried out with clients lying face upward on a table or mat. Sessions range in length and average about 45 minutes. Clients can receive treatment clothed or with direct touch to the abdominal areas. Chi Nei Tsang is part of a larger Healing Tao system to better educate people to better care for themselves.

Everyday Chi Kung

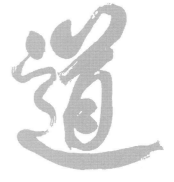

CHAPTER TEN

Chi Kung in Everyday Life

氣功

A great teacher once said that if what you learned on the "mountain top" cannot be applied at the bus stop, then you never really learned it. It is the true sage, the "wise one," who can take what they learn in their moments of meditation and enlightenment and integrate it into everyday life. Yet this "sage" exists within each of us. It is that part of us that can look at our lives in a holistic way, learning to move away from the illusion of form and get down to the essence of things.

This is the key to applying Chi Kung's basic principles to everything we do in life. We know in our hearts that when we are "in the moment" we have a sense that everything is as it should be. At these times we can see clearly where we are in the flow of things and it is easy to find solutions to apparent challenges. Chi Kung provides the set of tools that we can use at will to regain this sense of balance.

Waiting to get to the "mountain top" would severely limit the times we could create the ideal situations to practice Chi Kung, so modern life asks us to seek the sage-like approach. What sets the "master" apart is that they have learned the secret that each of us can map the principles of Chi Kung onto even the most mundane tasks in our daily lives.

The fundamentals of deep, diaphragmatic breathing, slow and intentional movement, and conscious visualization of the flow of Chi become part of everything we do. Imagine something you do everyday, such as getting into your car. It is usually a relatively mindless process of grabbing your keys, pulling open the car door, and driving off as soon as possible. Your mind is usually thinking about something else, such as where you need to be or what you will be doing over the weekend. In Chi Kung terms, this would be considered a way in which you are dissipating or weakening your Chi; whenever your focus is not on what you are doing, you are "giving away your Chi." This leads to frustration, anger, and general low energy.

Imagine instead an exercise in applied Chi Kung. When you reach for your car keys, you take a deep breath in, pulling your hand with the keys close to your body. Your steps to the car are slow and deliberate, linking a breath with each step. Exhale deeply as you insert the key into the lock and turn it. Inhale as you pull out the key and open the door. Exhale as you guide your body into the driver's seat, bringing your focus to your lower Tan T'ien, remaining conscious of your balance and shifting weight. Inhale as you hold the key, exhale as you put the key in the ignition and turn it. Feel your connection to the car, sensing it as an extension of your very being. Pause for a moment before shifting into gear, aligning your posture, and relaxing your shoulders and muscles right down to your toes. Smile from deep within and gather all your senses into a coherent focus. Fully present, this piece of practical Chi Kung has just shifted the whole matrix of your Chi and state of mind.

In China, Chi Kung masters apply their Chi balancing skills to a myriad of practices such as acupuncture, calligraphy, music, Kung Fu, emitted Wei Chi healing, feats of skill, and even dancing. It is understood that Chi Kung is not just reserved for those precious minutes of morning or evening exercise, but is a basic set of life principles that can enhance every aspect of our lives. Better health, greater joy, and a feeling of connection with all around us is the reward.

24-Hours-a-day Chi Kung

This describes a state where your energy is running correctly at all times. It is in your conscious awareness and under your control. Your energy operates all of the time—from the moment of conception through every moment of your life. When it stops working, so will you. When you stop what you are doing and practice Chi Kung, you take a special time to focus your attention. This is the only way to learn. The practices in this book give you a range of possible ways to do this.

However, once you have learned these or other practices, they become part of how you know and experience yourself. They change the relationship between your mind, body, and spirit, bringing them into a more fully integrated whole. You know what your energy system is, how it works, what it is doing, how to read it, and how to bring it back into correct alignment and balance.

Carrying out a specific practice for a particular purpose is a desirable and necessary thing. But there is a way in which you can also have your energy running, at a somewhat lower level, all of the time. This is called 24-hours-a-day Chi Kung. This does not require stopping what you are doing, but it does require paying attention so that your energy is in your consciousness and under your control. After a time, not only do you experience your energy as being *within* yourself, but also experience it *as* yourself. In fact, it becomes who and what you are. You become energy experiencing itself.

HOLDING ON TO YOUR CHI

It is also necessary to become aware of what to avoid—the situations, places, people, and events that will drain energy out of you, if you let them. Traveling in the rush hour, sitting on a subway, being in the middle of vast crowds of people, they can all be draining. In these situations there is nothing to do but protect yourself. Draw your external energy, your Wei Chi, tight around you like a protective coat and seal your energy in, but do not take any external energy into you. Slowly circulate the Microcosmic Orbit (*see* page 99.) Conserve and protect your energy as you would your wallet or purse.

If you encounter a person who drains you, either because they need your energy for themselves or because they are attempting to rob you of it, then again draw in. Do not give it away or let it be taken. Be aware of how this feels and happens, and avoid or minimize such encounters in the future. In the same way, avoid places that drain your energy. There is good energy and bad energy of location. Some places can even be dangerous. Learn to identify the difference and stay away from places that do not nourish or feed you, keeping your own environment as clear, clean, fresh, and uncluttered as possible. A few stalks of wild grass in a vase against a white wall can be exquisite.

Remain aware of the dynamics of the events and situations that you are involved in. It is not always possible to control events, but you can often decide whether or not to engage in them. In extreme cases, this may involve changing a job, moving somewhere else, or ending a relationship.

When you practice 24-hours-a-day Chi Kung your energy is working all the time. Food and diet are important aspects of this. Taoists consider that generally we eat too much. In its natural state the body can get by quite adequately on one meal a day—it has evolved to do so. Periodic fasting to cleanse out any accumulation of toxins and waste is also essential. Do this, at the very least, once in the spring and once in the fall. If you are not familiar with how to fast in a safe and controlled way, then seek advice and supervision from a health professional such as an Oriental Medicine practitioner or a naturopath.

With enough Chi Kung practice you can just draw in energy as a natural event. Your mind can read and modify your Chi as required. When you move or act you can do so in ways that preserve and accumulate energy. With 24-hours-a-day Chi Kung you can lead a busy, productive day—and end it feeling refreshed and relaxed.

24 Hours, 12 Meridians

In the West, we measure our days by dividing them into 24 hours. This is simply a convention we agree on in order to interact together. Each hour is divided into 60 minutes and each minute into 60 seconds.

It is usually a delicious delight, reserved for holidays, vacations, and days off, to "lose track of time," to not know what hour of the day it is. But there is also a way of knowing time through the energy system. The superficial Chi circulation runs in a continuous loop around the body, progressing from one channel and organ to the next in a strict sequence (*see* page 66). The Chi surges round our bodies in a 24-hour cycle, as if mirroring the Earth's rotation, and this acts as an internal metronome timing all of our biological functions. If we understand this circulation and what it affects and when, then we can align ourselves with our own natural internal rhythms. It is a way to synchronize with your natural biological cycles and so maintain better health. The Chi peaks in each of the 12 meridians for two hours each, and at these times it has an emphasized effect on the corresponding organ/function/official.

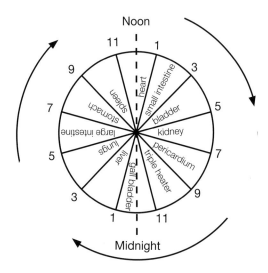

7am–9am   **Stomach/Earth/Yang**

This is the beginning of the day for most people. The first activity is to take food into the stomach, providing the energy to proceed through the day. Eat a wholesome breakfast. Some say it should be the biggest meal of the day.

In Oriental anatomy and the Table of Correspondences, the spleen also includes the pancreas. The relationship of this to the food that was taken in between 7a.m. and 9a.m. is self-evident. The food has to be digested using pancreatic secretions, and the energy contained in the food goes to the spleen. The spleen also controls the mind, so for many people this is the best time for study, thinking, and writing.

11am–1pm   **Heart/Fire/Yin**

The heart is the supreme controller, the Sovereign, and is a Fire Element. It comes to prominence at noon, when the Sun is at its zenith. This is the peak of the day, and the peak of your Fire. It is a time when you may be at your most active and get most things done. It is also a good time to interact with people. Most people eat lunch at this time, but it is advisable to eat lightly.

1pm–3pm   **Small Intestine/Yang/Fire**

The small intestines are involved in the digestion of the food taken in at breakfast and lunch. Blood is drawn to them. If you have eaten a big lunch you will tend to feel sleepy at this time. The function of the small intestine is to separate the pure from the impure, to take in what the body needs and to leave what it will eventually expel. This is also true on a mental level in deciding what is good for you and what is not.

3pm–5pm   **Bladder/Water/Yang**

The bladder is the controller of water. It is the sac-shaped organ that holds the waste liquids that will be excreted during the day. It corresponds to the late afternoon, when we are preparing for the night-time. In winter it is dusk, a time to begin to draw in. On a normal working day, people are preparing to leave work.

5pm–7pm   **Kidneys/Water/Yin**

The kidneys' primary function is to filter the fluids of the body. They separate the thick fluids from the thin. The thick fluids are retained and recycled in the body to provide the essential secretions that make everything flow correctly—such as saliva, tears, synovial fluids, and mucus. The thin fluids are passed to the bladder for elimination. This is the time of withdrawal from the day.

7pm–9pm   **Pericardium/Fire/Yin**

The pericardium is a sac that surrounds and protects the heart. It is also known as the Heart Protector. The pericardium has the important function in Oriental anatomy of protecting the heart, the supreme controller, from external insult and injury. It is like a Prime Minister in relation to a Sovereign. This is a time of relaxation, of protection. It is when we are usually at home, perhaps with family and loved ones.

9pm–11pm **Triple Heater/Fire/Yang**

The Triple Heater is a regulatory function in the body. It is not an organ, but has such significance in Oriental anatomy, that it is given the status of an organ. If the Triple Heater is out of order it can lead to excess activity—the fire flares up. This may be why some people get a "second wind" at this time, becoming active and staying up too late. This is a time to prepare to sleep and it is also the most common time of sexual activity—a definite Fire function. In the West we tend to stay up at night because of electric lighting and the television, but imagine or recall this time of the day if you were camping in the wilderness.

11pm–1am **Gall Bladder/Wood/Yang**

The gall bladder is generally seen as an extension of the liver. It collects secretions from the liver as bile, which is then passed into the small intestines to help digest fats. The gall bladder is constantly involved in the process of regulating the excretion of bile, and is therefore said to be the decision-maker. The top of the Gall Bladder channel runs over the sides of the head, and therefore affects the brain. At this time, we should now be asleep with our head on a pillow, so this may be the body's way of regenerating and refreshing the brain itself.

1am–3am **Liver/Wood/Yin**

The liver has many functions. It is like a chemical factory, involved in the processing of blood and fluids. It converts one substance into another, and neutralizes poisons and wastes. It is the largest single organ in the body, except for the skin. The liver can be viewed as the body's General, involved in planning or organizing. During this time a person is usually asleep. Any disturbance in the liver caused by the emotions of anger or frustration, and by drinking alcohol or other stimulants, can lead to disturbed sleep. This can be a major cause of insomnia.

3am–5am **Lungs/Metal/Yin**

The lungs are the organs involved in taking the fresh energy of the Heaven—oxygen—into the system and expelling carbon dioxide. As the Metal Element they control purification and letting go. Again, for most people this is still the time of sleep and dreams—those nocturnal excursions of the mind and consciousness. The lungs need to function correctly at this time. Any disturbance in respiratory function—because of a cold or flu, for instance—can disturb sleep.

5am–7am **Large Intestine/Metal/Yang**

The large intestine's major function is to collect the waste products of food in order to eliminate them from the body, and to re-absorb salts and fluids. As a Metal function it also relates to purification and letting go. During the night the bowels have accumulated the residue from food and digestion, and upon awaking it is common to empty the bowel. Unreleased or unexpressed sadness or loss can result in bowel dysfunction.

Waking Up

Waking up is a special time. You emerge from a state of sleep into a state of conscious awareness. At the point of awakening you are poised between two states, and this is reflected in your brainwave patterns where you are balanced between the Delta brainwaves of the deep subconscious through the Theta brainwaves of the subconscious and the Beta brainwaves of the conscious thinking mind via the Alpha rhythms. You are poised between consciousness and sleep. At this point you are able to access all states. If you have been dreaming, you can reflect on the dream and its significance, or you may have insights into thoughts, feelings, and events before the activities of the day begin. Take advantage of this time.

WAKING UP AS AN INSPIRATION

It is a good idea to set this time aside to use for your own self-awareness. If possible, set your waking time 15–30 minutes earlier than you need in order just to get up. Often you will obtain insights not available at any other time of the day. It helps to use the snooze button on an alarm clock, so that you can drift in and out of sleep without worrying about oversleeping. Take this as a time of reflection, learning, insight, and preparation for the coming day—whatever it may bring. Observe yourself and your mind.

Often, if you have been thinking about a specific issue or a problem, you may find the answer upon waking. This is often referred to as "sleeping on it." It is used in activities such as creative writing, in which one writes the night before and re-reads and edits the following morning. You may have had a conversation or discussion the previous night, and when you awake you have the answer or new insights. However, it is important not just to focus on your mind or feelings, but also to focus on your energy. Your energy is what drives everything and makes it work. This is the bottom line and the starting point.

ACTIVATING YOUR CHI

You can use this time to activate your Chi energy, to get ready to begin the activities of the day. The following Nei Dan exercise uses the mind to move the Chi.

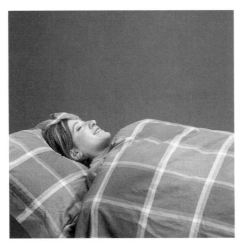

When you first wake up you can begin the day in the right way by smiling at yourself.

Practice

1   Smile at your organs as you would smile at a child or a loved one. Welcome them to the day. Give them your best wishes. Make sure they are doing all right and feeling good.

2   While still lying in bed, organize your energy. Begin by focusing on your navel. Slowly and carefully draw a Pa Kua there. Gently open it up by spiraling out and then back in again. Focus your Chi into your center, the navel, and gather and collect it there. Place the center of both palms, the Laokung point, over the navel. Left hand first for men, right hand first for women. Draw the heavenly Chi down into the navel and hold it there.

3   With your hands lying out to the sides with palms facing upward, use your mind to run Chi through the energy channels. As you breathe out, move the Chi from the torso down the inside arms to the fingers, and as you breathe in run it up the outside of the arms to the head.

4   Next, as you breathe out, run the Chi from the head down the side and the back of the body to the feet. When you breathe in again, draw the Chi from your feet up the inside of the legs and front of the torso back to the chest again.

5   Repeat this at least three times. End by returning to the navel. You have now activated your whole organ system in preparation for the coming day.

6   When you stand up, take the time to check your energy. Do the Energy Shower practice or the Three Tan T'ien to stimulate your system. Open the central channel of the Thrusting channel (Chong Mo), and make sure it is clear. Open and circulate the Eight Extraordinary meridians. Bring external Chi of Heaven and Earth into you. Stay focused in your center place.

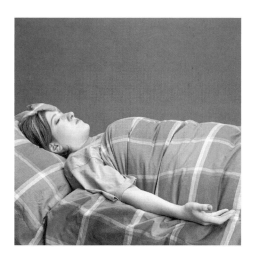

There are many practices you can do first thing in the morning. The one you choose to use may depend on a number of factors—what you know, the amount of time available, where you are, what else is going on (such as getting kids to school, and other people getting ready for work). It may not be possible to practice every morning. What is important is that you get into the habit of paying attention to your energy on waking up, and getting it activated and in order before launching into the new day.

Of course, this all presumes you lead a regular life. It may be that you wake in all kinds of situations—while traveling, in strange beds, on somebody else's couch or floor, in a foreign country, or at different times of the day or night. Maybe you stayed up late, worked through the night, were on the night shift, or had too much to eat or drink the night before … However, the overall principle remains the same. Give yourself time to awaken, clear your mind, and then organize your energy before launching into the day. Indeed, it is perhaps when you are in unfamiliar or stressful situations that it is best to use such practices. It will help you to deal and cope with the demands and stress of the different context.

For the last fifteen years I have taught a class on Tuesday mornings at 7am—a "Before Work" class. For an hour and a half people sit and go through a practice sequence of the Eight Extraordinary meridians. Then they go off to work or begin their day. Tuesdays seem to be one of the best days of every week.

Chi Kung at Work

At the beginning of the 21st century, many of us have discovered that the workplace has become the central focus of our lives. Work-related stress and stress-related illness are on the increase, creating severe impacts on our personal well-being, as well as on a wider scale. We need to find and regain a sense of balance and harmony in our daily professional lives. The art of Chi Kung practiced in the workplace is a simple, practical solution.

Although technology originally promised us much in the way of greater convenience and leisure, that promise is still unfulfilled. It seems that more and more time and personal energy are required for us to keep up with the demands of our jobs and professions. In fact, the increase in productivity and cost effectiveness are more than offset by the demands of the workplace on our personal time, attention, and energy.

When we add to this the growth of global competition, rapid organizational change, and relentless information overload, we have a picture of the contemporary workplace—a gigantic incubator of stress. A number of research studies into stress at work have shown that a large percentage of workers believe that their workloads are excessive; they worry about their job security, and they struggle to maintain a healthy balance between their work and personal lives. The American Institute of Stress estimates that 75–80 percent of all visits to physicians are precipitated by stress. This problem is not restricted to North America. In fact, a United Nations report in 1992 described job stress as "the 20th century disease." In Japan, the problem of workplace stress has become so severe that the Japanese have actually coined a term for it—the word *karoshi* means "to die at your desk."

The medical, economic, and emotional costs resulting from stress-related problems at work are alarmingly high for companies and employees alike. Ordinary stress management solutions such as jogging, working out at a health club, and meditation tend to be practiced before or after the working day. While these are certainly helpful, what is really needed is something that can be used by the individual at the actual moment of acute stress in the working day, to help regain a sense of mental and physical balance and harmony. This remedy should also support and enhance the employee's ability to remain calm, focused, and productive in their job. Chi Kung techniques provide the ideal solution to this.

CHI KUNG PRINCIPLES IN THE WORKPLACE

Chi Kung in the workplace involves taking responsibility for one's daily personal energy management. These principles include:

- Conserving energy—consistent reduction of unnecessary tension and energy loss.
- Condensing energy—rapid recharging and refreshing of oneself.
- Circulating energy—effective communication, cooperation, and teamwork.

- Refining energy—gaining clear mental focus, and greater intuitive intelligence.
- Projecting energy—leadership and interpersonal skills.

These principles are the basis of Chi Kung corporate stress management training and Executive Chi Kung® programs offered by Aspen Consulting Associates in the US, an innovative program pioneering Chi Kung in the workplace.

Effective application of Chi Kung in the workplace requires an understanding of these principles, techniques, and their proper application. For example, from a Chi Kung and Oriental medical perspective, stress is considered as body-energy that is rigidly bound-up, or in some way unbalanced. One frequent result of continuous, unmitigated stress in the workplace is coronary disease, an example of the Chi in the heart and arterial system becoming too "hot" or stagnant. In order to remedy this, it is necessary to "cool" the internal organs by discharging toxic energy and increasing internal Chi and blood circulation within the heart and between other internal organs. This internal organ "cooling" and rebalancing has positive effects on both the mind and body, producing greater mental clarity, intuition, and physical vitality.

CONSERVING AND INCREASING YOUR ENERGY AT WORK

Here are two simple and effective techniques you can use at work to conserve your energy and quickly recharge yourself.

Chi Kung Stagnant Energy Reduction Exercise

1 In a standing position, with feet shoulder-width apart and parallel, raise your arms above your head, inhale and rise up on your toes, gently stretching your whole body.

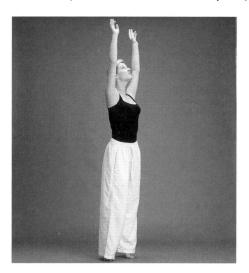

2 Hold this position for a moment and then quickly release the stretch; exhale and allow your arms, torso, and head to drop rapidly toward the ground. As you do this, drop your heels so that they strike the ground gently but firmly.

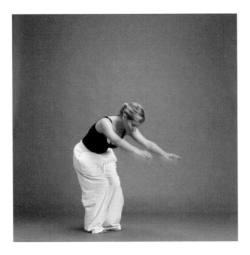 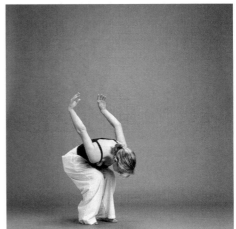

3 Visualize all the tension and stress in your body flowing into the ground through your feet.

4 Repeat this 3 or 4 times and then move into a squatting position with your palms touching the ground.

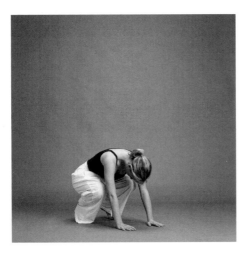

5 Visualize yourself absorbing clean, fresh energy from the Earth.

1 Stand in a normal standing position, with feet shoulder-width apart and parallel, knees slightly bent, with your arms hanging next to, but slightly away from, the sides of your body. You should feel that your armpits are slightly open (as if you were holding an egg in each armpit).

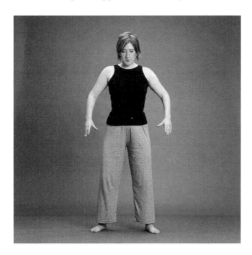

2 Visualize yourself as if you were standing as a skeleton or stick figure, concentrating on the bones within your body.
3 As you slowly and gently inhale, visualize energy being absorbed and condensing into the skeletal structure.
4 At the end of the inhalation, hold the breath for a moment and then slowly and gently release your exhalation. (Only visualize the energy condensing as you inhale. Rest on the exhalation.)
5 Repeat this sequence 6–9 times, briefly resting between inhalation and exhalation cycles.

Chi Kung at Leisure

Many activities are natural Chi Kung. Many things that people do inherently can function to activate the energy system. They are natural and spontaneous expressions of the body's energy. What is your Chi Kung? What do you already do that has an effect upon your energy system? How could you experience your energy more by changing your attention and focus? Try paying attention to what you already do, and observe your energy. Some common activities include:

Walking
Simple walking has powerful effects upon the energy. When you walk you breathe more deeply, and take in the outside air. Most people spend the majority of their time indoors, where the quality of the air degrades. A brisk walk will draw fresh heavenly Chi into you. When you walk you are upright and your feet are in contact with the ground—this activates the Yungchuan/Bubbling Spring point in the center of the soles. The movement of the hips activates Gall Bladder 29 and 30, which are powerful centers of Chi. The rhythmic alternate swinging of the hands and feet brings Chi into the extremities. If you do not have to drive or take a bus, then walk.

Gardening
Many people garden. Some have vast estates and elaborate gardens designed by landscape artists, some have an area around their house, and some have window boxes and indoor plants. In China there are many public parks landscaped according to Feng Shui principles. Outdoor gardening brings direct contact with the primary Earth. You stand between Heaven and Earth. Having your hands in the soil does you good, and you draw in energy through the Laokung points in your hands. Working with and caring for live plants is an interaction with their fresh, live, energy. Similarly, fresh, home-grown food, straight from the ground, is self-evidently preferable to canned and preserved goods.

Swimming
Swimming involves floating in water. You are horizontal rather than vertical, and your body can move up and down. This is a relief to the muscular and nervous systems, and it induces relaxation. A "flotation tank," which fully supports the body and in which there are no external stimuli, creates a profoundly deep and relaxing experience. But swimming involves the rhythmic movement of the arms and legs, and this distributes and equalizes the energy channels that run up and down the limbs. It puts the center of focus on the abdomen, centered on the navel. It is especially good for older people, as it relieves pressure on the joints. Swimming also activates the fluids in the body, which comprise a large portion of our bodily constituents. This is how we all began, floating in the amniotic fluid.

Many other exercises or sports activate and affect the energy system. Bike riding, running, tennis, dancing, soccer, and skiing, to name but a few, can all be seen to have energetic dimensions. When people engage in these activities, they work off the stagnant energy accumulated from work, while redressing their biological animal nature. Most such activities re-activate the Jing level of energy.

Any activity that you do can be Chi Kung, can be a form of practice. It all depends on what you do, and how you do it. Now that you have an awareness of what your energy system is, how it works, and what it feels like, pay attention to what you do, especially with activities that you perform on a regular and repetitive basis. Sitting in a chair can be Chi Kung practice, standing upright can be Chi Kung, walking across a room can activate your energy, shopping can be an energy-accumulating event. It all depends on what level of attention, awareness, and intent you apply.

Chi and the Environment

Your environment has a very powerful effect on your energy—contrast the difference between being in the middle of traffic downtown in rush-hour with standing on a hill top in the summer Sun with a fresh breeze on your face. This awareness of the energy of the environment is a refined art in China, with certain practitioners specializing in nothing else. This is known as Feng Shui—Wind and Water. The following is an introduction to the history, theories, and principles of this art, and its relationship to the Pa Kua.

THE FENG SHUI MAZE

There are many schools of Feng Shui, they have very little in common with each other, and they all claim to be the most effective. Feng Shui started in western China with the "form" school around A.D.600 and eventually moved southeast and evolved the "compass school" around A.D.700. The reason the compass school evolved is because western China has very interesting topography but southeastern China is mostly flat, so the compass directions became more important than the local topology. Nowadays, a good Feng Shui practitioner knows both schools. From these two schools, all the other schools evolved.

The schools can be likened to different levels of education. The intuitive, common sense school can be equated with a kindergarten, the "Black Sect" with middle school, the "Eight Direction" school with high school, and the "Flying Star" school with post-graduate work. They are all legitimate approaches and they represent different levels of complexity. The more complex compass schools look down on the simple schools, maintaining their

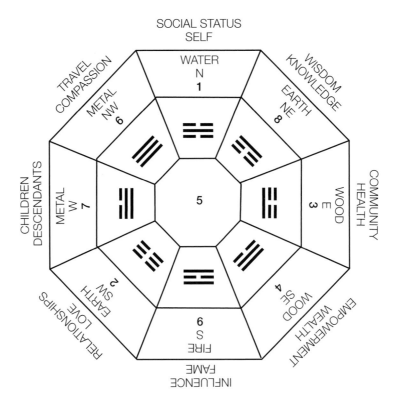

The Feng Shui Pa Kua

methods as simplification to the point of falsification. And the simple schools regard the compass schools as being unbearably cumbersome and so overly complex as to be utterly stifling. Neither of those extremes recognize the legitimacy of the "Eight Direction school," and so it goes …

The "Intuitive" school mostly deals with good, common sense interior decorating, based on principles of Taoism and Chi Kung. There are those who think it should not be called Feng Shui at all.

The Black Sect is the predominant form practiced today. It was invented by Professor Lin Yun in 1989 and is based on Tibetan Buddhist shamanic practices. This is mostly a "form" school that utilizes the eight direction influences in a unique way. For instance, they maintain that while standing in the doorway of any house or room, the right-hand corner relates to marriage and the left-hand corner relates to career. They recommend cures based on what they find in those areas. There is also a strong emphasis on ritual and spiritual influences as expressed in their house purification and door guardian rituals.

The "Eight Direction" school originated in Hong Kong and this school divides a house into eight locations: N, NE, E, SE, S, SW, W, and NW. Each location resonates with an aspect of life. Such as:

Social Ranking	North
Intellect	Northeast
Family	East
Wealth	Southeast
Fame	South
Romance and Marriage	Southwest
Children	West
Benefactors	Northwest

An offshoot of this compass school emphasizes the seven portents. These are auspicious or inauspicious areas of the house, as determined by the direction the front door faces. With this school, the energy of the inhabitants is also taken into consideration and this is determined by their energy composition at the moment of their birth.

The "Flying Star" school is by far the most complex of the compass schools and, according to them, they are the traditional system. This school emphasizes the age of the house. Every house built in a certain twenty-year period will have a similar energy arrangement. Once you factor in the direction it faces, then take into account the energy of the year and month and that of the inhabitants, you get a pile of energies in the same area that is said to reveal numerous details about all aspects of the people's lives. If an energy pile in any of the nine areas of a house or room is inauspicious, as it often is, they use fundamentally the same remedies as the other schools to cure it. Since the influence of the year and month are constantly changing, the practitioners are constantly having to make adjustments.

Presently, these are the major schools of Feng Shui. They are all legitimate but quite different one from another, so be sure to ask your practitioner which school they belong to so you will know what to expect when given a reading.

The table on page 164 describes some of the characteristics of each Kua, or trigram. Although in simplified form, you may find insightful ideas or intriguing hints for how to understand aspects of your own environment.

The North is the trigram Water.	Water is related to wisdom and danger.	The three gods (Happiness, Prosperity, and Longevity) are used to activate this area.
The Northeast is the trigram Mountain.	Academic success is the major concern here.	To activate this area, books may be placed in this area.
The East is the trigram Thunder.	The family is emphasized here.	To activate this area, plants are used or anything that branches out.
The Southeast is the trigram Wind.	This area is associated with wealth.	To activate this area, a three-legged toad with a coin in his mouth is often used. Bats attached to a string of coins are also used because their name fu also means good luck.
The South is the trigram Fire.	This location can bring fame or gossip.	To activate this area, red objects are used.
The Southwest is the trigram Earth.	The Earth represents the mother and marriage.	To improve your love life, a picture of a pair of mandarin ducks is traditionally used.
The West is the trigram Lake.	This area represents descendants.	To activate this area, a statue of the goddess Kuan Yin (who brings babies) was used.
The Northwest is the trigram Heaven.	This trigram represents the father or the Emperor.	To activate this area, a chain of five emperors was used.

Sleep

Sleep is the time when we turn everything "off" and enter into a state of recharge. It is a necessary function of all biological beings, and is a direct reflection of the rotation of the Earth around its axis, and the rotation of the Moon around the Earth, giving us the Day/Night Yang/Yin cycle. This alternating cycle affects and drives our energy in very specific ways.

In a natural state, without electric light, we would sleep when it goes dark and wake up when it gets light—we would be perfectly synchronized with the natural cycles. The normal pattern involves sleeping for about eight hours a night, one third of the day. Babies sleep longer, older people less. This is the time to reset the energy system and to allow the natural circulation to recharge itself. For most people this eight-hour period spans across the two-hour periods of circulation in the following channels based on Sun time.

Triple Heater	9pm–11pm
Gall Bladder	11pm–1am
Liver	1am–3am
Lungs	3am–5am
Colon	5am–7am
Stomach	7am–9am

Preparing for Sleep

To prepare for sleep, focus on your energy, not on your thoughts. In order to clear your energy and return it to center and neutral:

1   Before lying down, cleanse any accumulated or stagnant energy out of the system by doing the Energy Shower (*see* page 91.)
2   When you lie down, lie on your back, focus on your breathing, and clear your mind.
3   Calm all the internal organ/officials and stabilize your emotions by doing the Healing Smile (*see* page 89.)
4   Form a Pa Kua at the navel, to establish your center there. Place your palms and Laokung points over your navel. Draw energy in and out there.
5   Touch the tip of your tongue to the roof of your mouth and slowly begin to circulate the Microcosmic Orbit (*see* page 99,) smoothing and equalizing your energy in the Governor and Conception channels, so equalizing all of the organs.
6   Balance your Chi between the Three Tan T'ien along the central Thrusting channel.
7   Equalize your energy in all of your centers and channels.
8   Focus on gentle full breathing.
9   Keep your mind empty and clear.

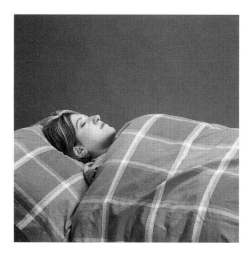

10 Tell yourself that you are going to allow your energy to slowly and gently circulate while you sleep.

11 Allow yourself to drift off.

If you wake up during the night, refocus on your energy system, putting it back into neutral. Do not chase thoughts or fantasies, but just allow them to come and go, observing them without becoming involved or connected with them. Stay focused, in center with your Chi. If you cannot go back to sleep, and there is nothing that you need to deal with, lie there with an empty mind and focus on your energy and breathing, using the time to recharge. If you are on night shift then you will be out of sync with the natural cycles, but the same principles of focusing on your energy apply.

Advanced practitioners of Chi Kung require less sleep than other people because they do not use the same amounts of energy as non-practitioners. Some do not sleep at all, but go into deep meditation while performing all of the usual regenerative functions that normally occur during sleep.

If you have a problem or illness in any of the organ/officials that are prominent during the night, then you may have disturbed or restless sleep. Likewise, if you are too excited, angry, sad, or worried—the emotional characteristics of the elements/organs prominent during night hours—then this will affect you. The best approach is to address the energy, not the emotion. Calm the energy down and the emotion will follow. If this is not something that you can do yourself, then seek professional assistance from an Acupuncturist or Oriental Medicine practitioner. Get your Chi operating correctly and all else will follow.

CHAPTER ELEVEN

Social Chi Kung

氣功

Babies and Children

Babies and young children naturally have good energy if nothing interferes with it before or after birth. They also do lots of natural Chi Kung—just watch them. They do, however, rely on the general energy field of their parents and extended family to protect them and keep their energy strong. Often, the best Chi Kung for young children is to reinforce that field and to make small, gentle adjustments to their energy-body to keep it as open and strong as possible, and to give them a good baseline to return to as they get older.

All children experience some stress, trauma, and shock to their energy systems as they grow up—their reaction to it reflects their constitution, temperament, and character, which are expressions of their energy-body. But while some wounding is inevitable, they can still come through it with their systems clear, open, and strong. Left to themselves and given good choices, they stay very healthy. They have an abundance of free Jing (physical energy) and, as documented in Chinese research, until about aged 18 months the energy center in their forehead is relatively open, so they can actually see past the material world. After that, it is supposed to "close" until they are about 12 years old to let them become grounded in the material world. So, how can we best support them?

In the womb, the developing child is held tight and protected; their whole world is a sense of ultimate closeness. When they are born, things change quickly. The physical umbilical cord to the mother is cut, but there remains an energetic one. The father holds his own larger sphere of protection and direct heart connection. The energetic cord to the mother is fully intact until the child reaches the teens. It is the job of the teenager to thin the cord and the job of the mother to let them. The cord should be totally severed by the mid-20s or there is unnatural over-dependence. They rely on the cord until they are 12–14 years old, when their personal energy field gets much stronger. It is important to remember that the parents cannot "feed" a balanced field to the child if they don't have one; because of this, Chi Kung for parents is of great benefit to children.

Newborn babies need to be swaddled; it provides the sense of protection they experienced in the womb. If this is not provided in some way, they pull in their field by closing their Dai Mo (Girdle channel) to achieve what they need, and this is not a good pattern to become comfortable with. Babies need closeness and the easiest way to achieve this is with a front-carrying pack for infants and a back-carrying pack for older children. Start them early (the first week). It is a way for both parents to "get close." This is not just body-close, but the parent's vibrant Heart/Chi, center Tan T'ien is enveloping, feeding, and calming them. If outside in windy weather, keep them close in your field when young—otherwise, again, they will close their Girdle channels to protect against the bombardment.

If you watch children, you will see that they need natural movement as well as closeness. The fewer "baby devices" you have, the better for the child. Playpens, walkers, and swings are particularly over-controlling if used too often. Children need to explore their world in safety, on their own—it keeps their energy flowing in the Eight Extraordinary meridians. Babies and children always go through a growth spurt of one kind or another after being on an extended nature outing because the energy of nature, the Chi-body of the Earth, literally feeds their field, just as it does in Chi Kung practice.

Children naturally do Chi Kung in play and non-competitive sports until they are around 12 years old. If they sit too often in front of a TV or computer (no matter what they are doing), they are not being active enough and their solar plexus area tends to close. Movies "imprint" images directly to the energy-body of the child, which they experience as being real because they are so permeable. Be careful what is "imprinting" on your child's field.

With divorce so prevalent today, many children move from one parent's home to the other. To help them adjust, spend a few extra moments at each change, consciously "shifting gears" with them. They have to disconnect from one field and reconnect with the next and they can use help with this. However, the mother-cord stretches as far as it needs to and many young children can perceive it.

In general, the best Chi Kung for children is early bonding with both parents (even if there is not a lot of "play"), and a loving, touching caregiver when they are absent. In addition, some gentle practices can help. A child that grows up with energy consciousness will naturally start to incorporate it into play and daily activity.

Harmonizing the Field

Native American mothers never put their children to bed without "smudging" them with sage or cedar to clear the day's events. Parents can do this with the energy of their hands by slowly moving them down the child's field (3–6 inches off the body) from head to foot. Use both hands, or one hand if you are holding the child, and do it front and back. This smoothes out the energy field; it is very relaxing, good for any stress, and children love it.

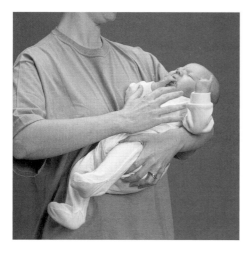

Tummy Rock

For stomach upsets in newborns or small children, move your hands back and forth in the field, 3–6 inches out, side to side over the abdomen.

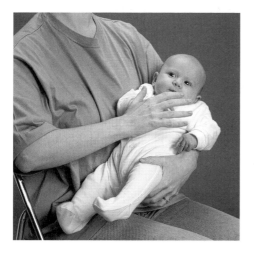

Solar Plexus Eye

With all babies and children, moving your hands clockwise over their solar plexus will greatly relieve general stress or the shock of any trauma or sports injury.

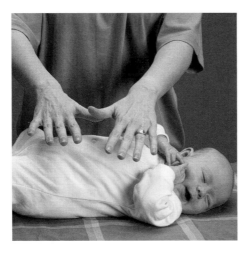

Solar Plexus Bowl

This is a good treatment to perform on children, gently on or off the body, for more serious stress. It helps them reset their energetic balance before habits set in. Teach them to do it themselves after they are 10–12 years old. (*See* page 140.)

Natural Regulation

Move your hands clockwise over the belly of a constipated child and counterclockwise over the belly of a child with diarrhea.

Chi Kung and Schools

Teaching Chi Kung in schools is a practical, simple, yet profound, program of preventive medicine that can be taught to schoolteachers, and then by them to their students. Such programs instruct in correct breathing and eating habits, relaxation techniques, regular and adequate exercise and body posture, control and harmony of thoughts and emotions, and the guiding light of human values—all of which are the essence of health and well-being.

Such programs can bring this knowledge to teachers, children, and parents, and to classrooms and homes through seminars, books, videos, games, and toys. The information is passed on to teachers through stress management seminars, and also there is instruction on how to teach these skills to the children. Other means by which children can receive this information include educational toys and games, and engaging parents' support through

Parent–Teacher Associations (PTAs). The benefits are many and include a healthier and more peaceful society, reduced stress among the teaching community, better quality of education, closer family ties, and billions of dollars saved in national healthcare.

THE SMART LIVING PROGRAM FOR SCHOOLS

Dr. Gaspar García, M.D., has created the Smart Living Program for Schools, in Marbella, southern Spain, a project that has created a cohesive program of preventive medicine, plus a practical mechanism for the transmission and implementation of this information in public and private schools. This innovative program serves as a model for Chi Kung in schools. Chi Kung in schools develops a broad spectrum of practical, conceptual, and behavioral abilities using a full range of innovative techniques

The conception of the program from a medical point of view (which follows WHO recommendations), and the far-reaching scope of the project, contrasts with the practicality and simplicity of its implementation, as well as the capacity to arouse interest within the teaching establishment. All of this gives the project the power to bring about true and deep health changes in society that will help millions of people to lead a healthier, happier, and more efficient life.

Objectives of the Smart Living Program
- To build a healthy, strong, and agile body, and attain a balanced mind and emotional development.
- To develop and maximize the potential of the diverse mental and psychological abilities, power of concentration, creativity, memory, coordination, sense of balance, flexibility, and relaxation.
- Discovery of the self as an integrated being—body, mind, and spirit. The experience of all possible positive and gratifying sensations. The practice of relaxation, concentration, and visualization. The experience of the "I" in complete harmony. The appreciation of the value *being* against *having*.
- To master the learned techniques and apply them throughout life as a useful tool in different situations, whether of a scholarly, personal, or social nature.
- To adopt healthy habits for life.
- The ability to open up to fellow people, to nature, and to the planet, resulting from a unity of the inner self.
- To maximize the application of human values through a true understanding of the natural laws of life and human relationships.
- The true final objective is to achieve a happy individual.

Chi Kung and the Elderly

The fastest growing population today is the elderly (those 65 and older). While the age parameters might be broad, it does define a population with unique and sometimes difficult health problems. When faced with the many transitions inherent to the ageing process, the challenge of maintaining balance and focus can seem overwhelming. As a method of self-cultivation, Chi Kung encompasses all facets of life, rejuvenating and restoring balance to the physical, emotional, and spiritual self, as well as improving health and increasing longevity

Altered status resulting from life-changing events, such as retirement or sudden chronic illness, can cause feelings of isolation and depression, directly impacting on mental health and productivity. A significant decrease in the physical demands of daily living, in addition to a lack of emotional or intellectual stimulation during this phase of life, often leads to inhibition, decreased spontaneity, and a loss of purpose. Many ailments commonly associated with the elderly can be attributed to this reduction in vital energy.

The beauty of Chi Kung is its accessibility to all, regardless of age and physical ability. Chi Kung forms can be modified to suit the required level of physical skill and mental focus. Instruction based on gentle, repetitive movement strengthens bones, increases balance, and improves memory and overall mental function. By using techniques of continuous motion, breathing, and meditation, the elderly learn to manage stress and improve emotional stability, thus promoting individual capacity for independent living.

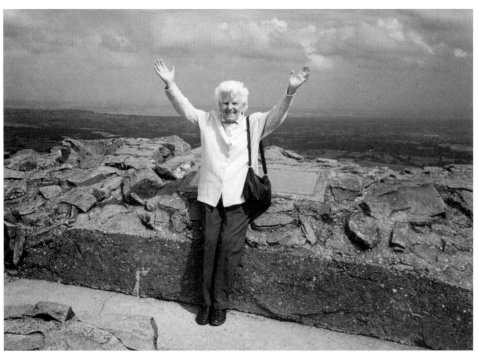

82 Years Old and on Top of her World

The simple, non-competitive nature of Chi Kung instruction nurtures self-exploration, self-expression, and mutual support. United in a sense of purpose focused on improved health outcomes, all things become possible. Because good health is related to a positive attitude, as healing is accelerated with the addition of Chi Kung exercise, natural compassion, creativity, and open-mindedness are reawakened.

A renewed sense of hope and purpose, resulting from this increased youthful energy, improves self-esteem, develops sociability, and leads to further self-empowering activities. Self-empowered individuals tend to become powerful leaders and role models for their families and communities. The basic technique of Chi Kung with its slow, no-impact movements makes it an ideal regime for the elderly.

BREATHING

The essence of Chi Kung is to rediscover one's natural breathing patterns. Internal Chi Kung exercises focusing on deep breathing and progressive relaxation can easily be performed in a lying or sitting position, making them particularly applicable to the elderly. Participants should be encouraged to become lost in their individual experience of Chi, focusing on feeling loose, while using the mind to direct and circulate healing energies.

The Essential (Abdominal) Breath
1   Sitting comfortably with the feet flat to the floor and looking straight ahead, rest the palms on the abdomen. Focus on relaxing this area of the body to allow free movement.
2   Breath in through the nose, allowing the abdomen to expand like a balloon as the diaphragm drops, massaging the internal organs. Relaxing the chest muscles, allow the rib cage and spine to expand, so filling the chest cavity.
3   Exhale slowly through the nose. Repeat, resting as needed.

Standing postures gently teach coordination of breath and movement, generate Chi, and greatly enhance strength, balance, and Chi flow throughout the body. This exercise can easily be modified for use in both a lying or sitting position.

Push Away Heaven, Push Away Earth

1   Standing comfortably erect, release the tension from the legs and hips by relaxing the spine and unlocking the ankle, knee, and hip joints. Relaxing the chest and abdomen, breath in slowly through the nose.

2   Slowly exhale, rotating the upper torso to the right and extending the left arm directly overhead, pushing the palm flat toward the ceiling while lowering the right arm and pushing the palm flat toward the floor. Make certain that the feet are flat to the floor and that the legs, hips, and waist are relaxed.

3   Inhaling slowly through the nose, relax and allow the body to rotate naturally to the left, while reversing the direction of the push. Exhale slowly as you push away Heaven—push away Earth. Relax and breath naturally, allowing the Chi to move from the tips of the fingers to the tips of the toes opening the complete side meridians. Repeat, focusing on coordinating breath and movement, resting as needed.

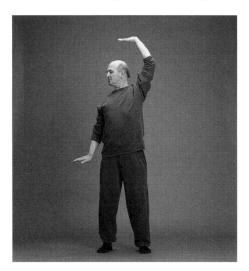 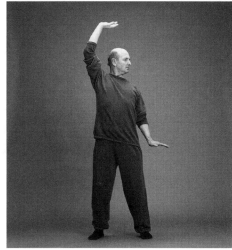

Self-massage is most effective when energy is abundant, following internal or external Chi Kung exercise. The mind plays a crucial role in guiding healing energy throughout the body.

Internal Organ Massage

1 Sit comfortably erect with the feet flat to the floor, looking straight ahead. Release the tension from the legs and hips, allowing the chair to support fully the weight of the body (do not push against the floor).

2 Forming a loose fist with the left hand, stimulate the nerve endings of the right hand by gently "pounding" the entire palm of the right hand. Relax the wrists and hands with exaggerated looseness. Breath as if you are doing no exercise.

3 Vary the point of pressure to stimulate all of the body's internal organs and functions.

4 Loosely lace the fingers together. Slowly rotate the wrists while relaxing the hands, gently massaging the spaces between the fingers.

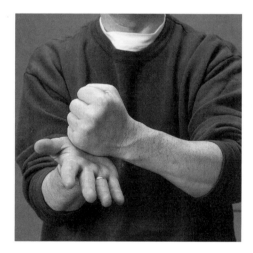 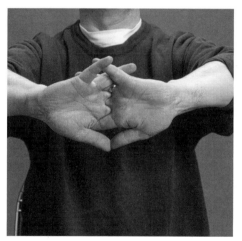

Chi Kung for Special Needs

Since Chi Kung uses very simple exercises to harness the natural energy inside and outside the body, it can be practiced by people of any physical or mental ability. To accommodate the varying range of abilities and disabilities, slight alterations can be made to the movement patterns without altering their effectiveness. People with physical disabilities, serious illnesses, frailty of old age, learning difficulties, high levels of stress, and those recovering from mental illness and substance abuse can all be helped by Chi Kung.

It may be obvious to say that people with special needs can be helped by Chi Kung, because it is a health practice that stimulates the body's own natural instinct to promote healing and well-being, but people with special needs are often deprived of the opportunity to learn and be guided in such practices. Their "special need" should be seen more as a need for access to teachers and information than as a need dictated by their particular disability. Happily, this imbalance is in the process of being redressed. Many excellent books on Chi Kung have been published in the West and many more classes have become available in hospitals, day clinics, and rehabilitation centers.

One of the most exciting aspects of Chi Kung for people with special needs is the fact that they can take total charge of themselves—mentally, physically, and emotionally—during the period of practice. This is, of course, true for anyone who practices Chi Kung, but for many disabled people there is very little in their lives that is totally within their own domain of control. They may depend on others to drive them from place to place, to wheel them, feed them, wash them, and toilet them. The infringement on personal dignity can be soul destroying. Also, there may be many other beneficial forms of exercise within a particular person's health program that it may not be possible to perform unaided. For instance, a man recovering from the effects of a stroke might need to have other people moving his limbs for him, or offering him other forms of physical support. With Chi Kung, no outside help is necessary and this means human dignity and personal power are truly honored.

Checklist

If you are a person with special needs and would like to begin to practice Chi Kung, you may wish to try any of the exercises described in this book. However, whatever you choose to do, please take note of the following checklist.

1   **Choose the best position. This may mean that sitting down is the best position for you, rather than standing. Be sure to have your back supported well and your feet in contact with the floor or a footstool. It may be that lying down might be best for you, and you may wish to have a small pillow under your knees. If getting up and down from the floor is difficult for you, lie on a sofa or a firm bed.**

2   **Be comfortable. Take special note of the temperature and be aware of any possible drafts. Have a blanket over you or keep one nearby in case you begin to feel chilled.**

You may even wish to start your session with some music if this will help you feel relaxed.

3 Common sense and medical advice. If you have participated for some time in your own healthcare decisions, you will have already found out if there are any particular kinds of movement or activity that may not be appropriate to your condition. If you are not sure, consult with those who have been helping you formulate your health practice. For instance, if you have arthritis, you will probably know that there are times in the cycle of symptoms when it is not advisable to move joints. At such times, it is possible to practice the visualization aspects of Chi Kung without the movement.

4 Feel your own power. Enjoy the feeling that during your time of practice you are totally in charge of what happens. No one will be doing something for you. You will be doing something for yourself.

Adapting Exercises

If you have a particular disability, you will have already learned many ways of adapting to your situation. When you consider how to do a particular Chi Kung exercise, simply apply this well-developed skill. If you are unaccustomed to doing movement patterns, try the following in order to demystify the process.

Deconstructing an Exercise

As you read a description of movement, or if you are watching a teacher, notice what each part of the body is doing separately—the left hand, the right hand, the head, and the legs. If you do not have movement in any particular part of your body, then imagine the movement.

Symmetry is on your Side

Even if you do not have full movement, or a symmetrical body shape, the exercises are developed in a symmetrical manner and so you can grasp their shape by looking at one side of the pattern at a time, or by moving one side of your own body at a time. If you have no movement on one side, imagine the movement.

Reconstructing an Exercise

When you come to put the whole pattern together, let your mind follow the whole movement process very slowly before you attempt to move. Practice in your mind before you practice with your body. In any case, most of what happens is down to the idea that is opened up in the mind. If you keep your mind open, the benefit of the exercise will come to you.

Developing your Energy with Partners and Groups

Once you have familiarized yourself with the reality of Chi energy, you can use it to work on friends, family, and colleagues. Try these simple exercises with a partner first. Once you have "connected" your energy with someone else's, you can try to expand the flow in a larger group. The power and collective energy that emanates through working with a group helps to increase each individual's Chi flow.

Exercise with a Partner

This exercise can either be practiced sitting or standing. The passive partner either stands or sits down with eyes closed and mind relaxed. The active partner should also take a little time to quiet the mind and relax the breathing. Focus your awareness to the lower Tan T'ien.

1   Focus your energy to the palm of the hands at the Laokung point.
2   Start by placing your palms at each side of your partner's head so that the Laokung point is facing them.
3   With a relaxed "soft" focus let the energy pass through your hands to your partner's head.
4   Staying relaxed and focused, proceed to let your palms move around your partner's body (without touching the body,) from the head downward, covering both the front and rear.
5   Try to "feel" through your hands any areas that you think will benefit from extra attention or focus.

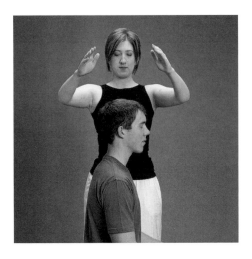
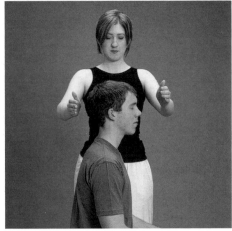

6 If you "feel" the need to hold the energy a little longer at a particular place, then do so.

7 Finish the practice by "washing down" your partner's face and body with your energy, from the top to the bottom.

When the session has finished allow a few minutes for your partner to "come to." Take some time to discuss how the session felt and any areas where your partner felt more or less benefit. Change roles and allow the other person to give you the treatment.

Exercise with a Group

Again, this exercise can be practiced either sitting or standing.

1 The group should form a circle with each person being no more than an elbow distance from the next.

2 Each member should take time to become aware of their connection to the Earth through the Yungchuan (Bubbling Spring) at the soles of the feet, and a connection to the Heavens through the Paihui point at the crown of the head.

3 Allow a few minutes to develop this connection.

4 With the arms hanging loosely by your sides, allow the hands, facing downward, to open softly and become aware of the energy in the palms.

5 When you have developed the feeling of energy in your palms, turn the left palm upwards, keeping the right facing down.

6 Move your hands to allow your right hand, facing downward, to be about 6 inches above that of the person on your right, and the left hand 6 inches below the person on your left, facing upward.

7 Hold this position for some time to allow the energy to flow through the group.

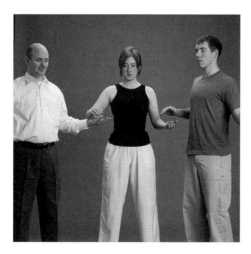

8 Synchronize the breathing pattern of the whole group, so that everybody is breathing in and out at the same time.

9 As you breathe in, draw the Chi into your left palm and up your arm to the center of the chest.

10 As you breathe out, send it from the center of the chest down the inside of the right arm down to the right palm.

11 Feel the Chi flowing from one side to the other, through you and through the whole group.

12 Finish the session by having each member of the group bring their hands up above their heads with the palms facing forward into the middle of the group.

13 Completing a circle out in front of you, allow your hands to move down to your lower Tan T'ien to rest for a few minutes.

When practiced with a soft "open" mind this exercise can help to increase the flow of energy through both the individuals and all of the members of the group. When you have finished, discuss the experience together.

Chi Kung—Healing for the World

One basic use of Chi Kung is that it enables our energy, and so our whole self, to flow naturally, and with a sense of healthy anticipation for the adventures of the future unfolding within and around us. This powerful purpose of Chi Kung can literally change the world, one central nervous system at a time, as it comes to be practiced by more and more people around the globe. Human evolution has not prepared us for the speed of change that the technological and communications revolution has unleashed on the planet, coupled with the rapidly changing demands of a population exceeding six billion people.

Chi Kung is in many ways a prescription for the future, as it was designed to enable the practitioner to flow with change in a more healthful and expansive manner. In the same way, the widespread practice of Chi Kung could end our healthcare crisis, reduce unemployment, diminish violence within society, and, ultimately, end war between societies, while at the same time enhancing creativity and productivity. If this sounds too good to be true, consider the following facts.

Medicine

Kaiser Permanente in California carried out a long-term study that showed that over 70 percent of illness requiring a doctor's attention is due to stress or psychosocial distress. Yet, medical research indicates that Chi Kung practice can easily, cheaply, and safely address many of these problems.

Violence

A Chi Kung program at Folsom State Maximum Security Penitentiary, California, has seen a reduction of violent incidents since implementing the program, with the reduction in some inmates as high as 70 percent. If Chi Kung can have this effect in Folsom prison, imagine what might happen if school children, families in crisis, and government leaders worldwide begin to practice these integrating and creative mind–body tools.

Unemployment and Stress

The Royal Academy of Paediatrics in the UK has found that households with high levels of stress produce children who are less employable as adults, making Chi Kung a tool for both families and schools to enhance our future workforce, in time lessening the demand on social services.

Creativity and Productivity

Stress is believed to cost US businesses upward of $300 billion per year, or $7,500 per employee per year, in lost productivity.

In 1999 an event called World T'ai Chi & Qigong (Chi Kung) Day was initiated to bring the vastly underutilized potential of Chi Kung into the public eye worldwide. You can find out more and become involved by contacting www.worldtaochiday.org. Each year, tens of thousands of people who have experienced the healing benefits of Chi Kung and Tai Chi conduct mass public exhibitions worldwide. The goal is to educate, promote global health, and to provide a model of cooperation across racial, ethnic, and geopolitical boundaries as humanity unites to celebrate an act of global health.

Your Life as an Energy Event

I hope that this book has given you an understanding and appreciation of the profound practices that are called Chi Kung. They will indeed give you Energy for Life. In the book we have looked at what Chi Kung is, where it came from historically, and examined the energy system—its anatomy and physiology. This was followed by basic Chi Kung practices that anybody in average health can do, and also some more advanced practices. Finally, we looked at how it can all relate to our normal everyday lives. The book is laced, and graced, with contributions from 22 leading practitioners. There are practices in this book that can last you a lifetime. You can build them into your ordinary life and do them every day.

The nature of language is such that we are able to communicate and share our experiences, feelings, and ideas together in a rich variety of ways. But from a Taoist and Chi Kung perspective there are absolute limitations where language ends and experience begins. Our energy is the foundation of our experience. By doing these simple practices you will experience yourself in new ways.

In the West, the energy part of ourselves has been missing from our history and our culture. But now with Chi Kung this is changing. Our view of ourselves and what we are is shifting focus. It is the answer to many questions. It has the power to transform our world.

There are always some principles and values that act as beacons in our lives, reference points by which we set our course. Some of these are personal to each of us, and some we share with others existing in our particular time and culture. However, some are beyond all of this—they are based upon our common humanity with all people of all times. They are part of what it means to be human.

In Chi Kung, the primary guiding principle and value is the understanding of our energy dimension. This involves recognition of the difference and interplay between our subjective internal feelings, awareness, wants, and needs, and the objective physical and energetic reality—the Yin/Yang balance of our integrated whole.

But the magic is that if we put our attention and time into our energy system, then many positive and desirable things automatically follow on. Chi Kung is a way to get your energy functioning correctly, to increase the volume, heighten the frequency, and put it under your conscious control. If you simply do the practices you will benefit physically, emotionally, mentally, and spiritually. If you focus on your life as an energy event, everything will be better. You will feel more complete and fulfilled. You will become One within yourself. You will be a great asset to those that you love and care for, and work and interact with. And you will contribute to a better world.

All of this, and much more, is available to you now. Everything you need is already inside you. It could not be simpler. All you have to do is practice. Practice Chi Kung and you will have energy for life.

My best wishes and very best Chi,
Jim MacRitchie

Information and programs of classes, training, and individual treatment at The Body-Energy Center are available on request. Contact details are:

The Chi Kung School,
The Body-Energy Center,
2730 29th Street, Boulder, CO 80301, USA

Tel: USA-303-442-3131
Fax: USA-303-442-3141
E-mail: jamesmacritchie@earthlink.net
Website: www.thebodyenergycenter.com

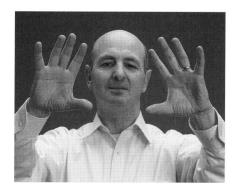

氣功 Appendices

About the Contributors

James MacRitchie

James MacRitchie is the principal author and general editor of this book. Originally from Liverpool, England, he lives in Boulder in the Rocky Mountains of Colorado. Jim co-directs The Chi Kung School at The Body-Energy Center with his wife, Damaris Jarboux. He has been in clinical practice of Acupuncture since 1977, and now specializes in Zhen Jou Chi Kung and teaches. He has three children, and aspires to live in accordance with The Tao.

Jim is Founder of the National Qigong (Chi Kung) Association * USA, Founding President of The Acupuncture Association of Colorado, and a Council Member of The World Academic Society of Medical Qigong, Beijing, China. He was Co-Founder/Director of The Natural Dance Workshop, London (1975–81) and The Evolving Institute, Boulder (1982–88). His previous books include *Chi Kung: Cultivating Personal Energy* (Element Books, 1993) and *The Chi Kung Way—Alive with Energy* (HarperCollins, 1997).

The following 22 teachers contributed the sections in the text credited to them. They are listed in the order of appearance in the book. These people are recognized Western leaders in the field of Chi Kung and while being widely experienced they are specialists in the topic they have written on. They bring to you a wealth of knowledge and expertise, contributing to this unique cross-section of all aspects of Chi Kung. Many of them are members of the

National Qigong (Chi Kung) Association * USA (NQA), the organization which they collectively created together. WASMQ is The World Academic Society of Medical Qigong. Their contact details are included here for you to reach them directly for further information.

PREFACE (PAGE XI)

Solala Towler

Solala Towler lives in Eugene, Oregon. He is the publisher of *The Empty Vessel, A Journal of Contemporary Taoism*, and is also the author of six books on Taoism including *A Gathering of Cranes* and *Embarking on the Way: A Guide to Western Taoism*, as well as the *Tao Paths* series. Solala is an instructor of several styles of Chi Kung and leads yearly tours to China. He has served as President of the National Qigong (Chi Kung) Association * USA.

The Abode of the Eternal Tao,
1991 Garfield Street, Eugene,
OR 97405,
USA

Tel: 541-345-8854
Fax: 800-574-5118
E-mail: solala@abodetao.com
Web site: www.abodetao.com

BUDDHIST CHI KUNG (PAGE 12)

Dr. Gaspar García, M.D.

Gaspar García is an M.D. and practicing acupuncturist. He is the President of the European Luohan Gong Federation and Vice-President of the WASMQ. He is considered the most advanced Luohan Gong master in the West and has introduced this system in Europe, the United States, and several Latin American countries. He is well-known for teaching children and school teachers and has created the Energy Management Program to manage stress.

Paseo de Colombia 172 A, Elviria,
Marbella, 29600, Málaga, Spain

Tel: 34-95-283-4471
Fax: 34-95-276-4305
E-mail: Gaspargarcia@ingenia.es
Web site: www.luohan.com and
www.salusline.com

INNER ALCHEMY AND SPIRITUAL DEVELOPMENT (PAGE 20)

Roger Jahnke

(See Meditation in Chi Kung *below*)

Roger Jahnke
(*See* Meditation in Chi Kung *below*)

MEDICAL SCIENCE AND RESEARCH (PAGE 25)

Kenneth M. Sancier, Ph.D.

Ken Sancier received a Ph.D. from Johns Hopkins University. He is Founder and Chairman of the Board of the Qigong Institute and a Professor at the American College of Traditional Chinese Medicine. He has published articles describing his scientific studies of the effects of Qigong on the body and reviewing Medical Qigong research. He developed the Computerized Qigong Database for searching the literature for Qigong research. Ken is widely regarded as one of the experts in the United States on the scientific basis of Chi Kung.

Qigong Institute,
561 Berkeley Avenue,
Menlo Park, CA 94025, USA

E-mail: matsu@nanospace.com
Web site: www.qigonginstitute.org

MEDITATION IN CHI KUNG (PAGE 83)

Roger Jahnke, OMD

Roger Jahnke has been in clinical practice as a physician of Chinese medicine since 1977. In 1967 he began the practice of T'ai Chi, Chi Kung (Qigong), and Nei Dan. He has traveled to China many times to explore the secrets of Qi in the hospitals, temples, and sacred sites. Roger is the Director of the Institute of Integral Qigong and T'ai Chi and the Chair of the Qi Cultivation Department at the Santa Barbara College of Oriental Medicine. He is author of *The Healing Promise of Qi* and *The Healer Within*. He is a Founding Board Member of National Qigong (Chi Kung) Association * USA and has served as Chairperson.

Institute of Integral Qigong and T'ai Chi,
243 Pebble Beach,
Santa Barbara, CA 93117, USA

Tel: 805-685-4670 and 800-824-4325
Fax: 805-685-4710
E-mail: rjahnke@west.net
Web sites: www.HealerWithin.com and
www.Qigong-ChiKung.com

Dennis Lewis

Dennis Lewis teaches Natural Breathing, Qigong, T'ai Chi, and Meditation, and is a Chi Nei Tsang practitioner. He is certified to teach Chi Kung and T'ai Chi by Taoist masters. Dennis is the author of the highly acclaimed book, *The Tao of Natural Breathing*, and the audio program *Breathing as a Metaphor for Living* (Sounds True). He is Co-editor with Jacob Needleman of *Sacred Tradition & Present Need*.

Authentic Breathing,   Tel: 415-282-4896
PO Box 31376,   Fax: 415-641-7716
San Francisco, CA 94131,   E-mail: info@authentic-breathing.com
USA   Web site: www.authentic-breathing.com

THE MICROCOSMIC ORBIT: SMALL HEAVEN MEDITATION (PAGE 99)

Dr. Russell DesMarais

Russell DesMarais is a Doctor of Chiropractic and an Acupuncturist. He has studied Qigong in China with Doctors and Masters. He was certified as an International Chi Kung Doctor and Master teacher through the National Science and Research Center for Applied Chi Kung in Benxi, China. He was Founder and Director of Turtle Island Health Center, St. Paul, Minnesota, USA and is a Past-President of the National Qigong (Chi Kung) Association * USA.

Three Rivers Crossing Qi Gong School,   Tel: 651-291-7700 and 651-291 7608
Turtle Island Health Center,   Fax: 651-291-7779
571 Selby Avenue, St. Paul, MN 55102,   E-mail: info@threeriverscrossing.com
USA   Web site: www.threeriverscrossing.com

THE MACROCOSMIC ORBIT: BIG HEAVEN MEDITATION (PAGE 102)

Richard Leirer

Richard is the Director of the Qigong Academy, in Cleveland, Ohio, and an instructor in T'ai Chi and Qigong. He began his training in 1972. He has received a Masters Certificate from the Chinese Qigong Society of Cleveland, and has had research on the benefits of Qigong T'ai Chi for Veterans suffering from P.T.S.D. published at the World Medical Qigong Conference, Beijing, China. He is the Founding Vice-President of the National Qigong (Chi Kung) Association * USA.

The Qigong Academy,
5553 Pearl Road,
Cleveland, OH 44129, USA

Tel: 440-842-9907
E-mail: RJL142@aol.com
Web site: www.QigongAcademy.com

LYING, SITTING, STANDING, MOVING (PAGE 104)

Jesse Dammann

Jesse Dammann teaches at The Chi Kung School at The Body-Energy Center, Boulder, Colorado, as well as offering personal training and instruction. He is a Founding Board Member of National Qigong (Chi Kung) Association * USA. Jesse specializes in researching the interconnections between many different styles of Chi Kung and the various manifestations of energy cultivation that have emerged in different cultures.

31876 Lillis Place,
Golden, CO 80403, USA

Tel: 303-642-9635 and 303-442-3131
Fax: 303-442-3141

THE EXTERNAL ENERGY FIELD (WEI CHI) (PAGE 121)

Russell DesMarais

(See The Microcosmic Orbit *above*)

THE FIVE ANIMAL FROLICS (PAGE 124)

John Du Cane

John Du Cane began Chi Kung in 1975. In 1990 he founded Dragon Door Publications, a resource for Qigong, fitness, and martial arts, including a regular catalog, *Vitalics,* and a publishing company. He is the author of four instructional videos on Chi Kung and a book on The Five Animal Frolics. He teaches seminars on a variety of Chi Kung methods, and promotes training and programs by a variety of teachers.

Dragon Door,
PO Box 4381,
St. Paul, MN 55104, USA

Tel: 651-645-0517
E-mail: dragondoor@aol.com
Web site: www.dragondoor.com

Michael Winn

Michael Winn is a Past-President of the National Qigong (Chi Kung) Association * USA. He has written six Chi Kung books with Mantak Chia, including *Taoist Secrets of Love: Cultivating Male Sexual Energy*. Michael is Founder of Healing Tao University, the largest Tao "Chi training" program in the West with 30 week-long retreats in New York's Catskill Mountains. His Tao Chi Kung Home Study Audio/Video courses are unique in their depth.

PO Box 601,   Tel/Fax: 973-777-4442 and 888-999-0555
Asheville, NC 28802, USA   E-mail: info@HealingTaoUSA.com
                                               Web site: www.HealingTaoUSA.com

OVARY AND TESTICLE BREATHING (PAGE 132)

Marcia Wexler Kerwit, MPH, Ph.D.

Marcia Kerwit has been teaching Healing Tao since 1983 and was honored in 1994 as a Senior Instructor. Marcia is a co-founder of the Women's Qigong Alliance. She specializes in women's practices and teaches internationally. She co-authored *Healing Love Through the Tao: Cultivating Female Sexual Energy* with Mantak and Maneewan Chia, and has written and co-authored other books on women's health including *A New View of a Woman's Body*.

Bay Area Healing Tao,   Tel: 510-834-1934
P.O. Box 10824, Oakland, CA 94610,   Web site: www.thewqa.org
USA

CHI KUNG HEALING (PAGE 136)

Damaris Jarboux

Damaris Jarboux has broad experience in both Eastern and Western medicine, and serves as a bridge between them. An R.N. since 1967, in private practice since 1986, she is Co-Director of The Chi Kung School at The Body-Energy Center in Boulder, Colorado. Trained in China and the West, she is a respected innovator and teacher, and has created numerous training programs, from self-practice and family care to advanced Chi Kung Healing. She is a Founding Board Member of the National Qigong (Chi Kung) Association * USA, and Chair of the Chi Kung Healing sub-committee.

The Chi Kung School
The Body-Energy Center,
2730 29th St, Boulder, CO 80301, USA

Tel: 303-447-0484
Fax: 303-442-3141
E-mail: damarisj@earthlink.net
Web site: www.thebodyenergycenter.com

MEDICAL QIGONG THERAPY (PAGE 142)

Dr. Jerry Alan Johnson, Ph.D., D.T.C.M., D.M.Q. (China)

Jerry Alan Johnson is licensed as a Doctor of Traditional Chinese Medicine in Beijing, China. He is Director and Founder of The International Institute of Medical Qigong in Pacific Grove, California; Dean of Medical Qigong Science and Director of the Medical Qigong Clinic at the Five Branches College of Traditional Chinese Medicine in Santa Cruz, California; and a Council Board Member of the WASMQ, Beijing, China. His section on Medical Qigong Therapy is excerpted from his textbook *Chinese Medical Qigong Therapy: A Comprehensive Clinical Text.*

The International Institute of Medical Qigong,
P.O. Box 52144, Pacific Grove, CA 93950,
USA

Tel: 831-646-9399
Fax: 831-646-0535
E-mail: drjerryalanjohnson@earthlink.net
Web site: www.qigongmedicine.com

CHI KUNG AS THERAPY (PAGE 145)

Adrian Lowe

Adrian Lowe has practiced and trained in his family art of LAMAS Qigong, which dates back to the Han dynasty, for almost 50 years, and is the world's leading authority. He is the Founder of the LAMAS Qigong Association, and The National Qi Gong College, UK, and has a private practice in Chi Kung Therapy, in Retford, Nottinghamshire, UK. He has produced two videos, *Wild Goose Qigong* (Daoyin style) and *LAMAS Tai-Chi Qigong*, and the book *The Art of Daoyin.*

National Qi Gong College, Chancery Lane,
Retford, Notts DN22 6EU, UK

Tel/Fax: 01777-700055
E-mail: info@nqc.ac
Web site: www.nqc.ac

Ron Diana

Ron Diana is a Senior Instructor and practitioner with the Universal Tao. He has studied Taoist Healing, Internal Alchemy, T'ai Chi, and Chi Kung with several Taoist Masters since 1973, most extensively with Mantak Chia and Dr. Stephen Chang. Co-author of *Chi Nei Tsang Internal Organ Massage* and *Bone Marrow Nei Kung*, both best-selling Taoist books, Ron teaches internationally and has a private practice in Chi Nei Tsang and Chinese Herbology in New York and New Jersey.

Tao Healing Arts,
1 Union Square West #815,
New York, NY 10003, USA

Tel: 212-242-1410 and1-888-291-5208
(pin 1642)
Fax: 212-242-2404
E-mail: taoarts1@aol.com
Web site: www.taohealingarts.com

Healing Tao of New Jersey,
1 Coles Crossing,
Hillsdale, NJ 07642, USA

Tel: 201-358-0620
Fax: 201-722-8934
E-mail: RHDiana@aol.com
Web site: www.Taohealing.com

CHI KUNG IN EVERYDAY LIFE (PAGE 149)

Francesco Garri Garripoli

Francesco Garri Garripoli, a longtime Eastern healing practitioner, is the author of *Qigong— Essence of the Healing Dance* and was director of the PBS television documentary *Qigong— Ancient Chinese Healing for the 21st Century* seen nationwide in the US and Canada on PBS. He and his wife, Daisy, perform in a series of Wuji Qigong instructional videotapes. His current project, WellRing, is helping to introduce Qigong into mainstream healthcare. See his websites to learn more.

Wuji Productions,
5172 Kahuna Rd,
Kapaa, Kauai
Hawaii, USA 96746

Fax: 508-464-5809
Web sites: www.wujiproductions.com and
www.wellring.com

CHI KUNG AT WORK (PAGE 158)

Gunther M. Weil, Ph.D.

Gunther Weil is an internationally recognized corporate consultant, educator, and Chi Kung teacher. He is the Founding Chairperson of the National Qigong (Chi Kung) Association * USA. Dr. Weil received his doctorate in social psychology from Harvard University. He is Co-director with his wife, Ellen Weil, of Aspen Consulting Associates LLC, offering customized executive retreats, leadership training, Cultivating Presence Intensives and Executive Chi Kung® programs to their international clients.

Aspen Consulting Associates LLC,
4337 County Rd 113, Carbondale,
CO 81623, USA

Tel: 970-945-4050
Fax: 970-928-8185
E-mail: weil@aspen-consult.com
Website: www.aspen-consult.com

CHI AND THE ENVIRONMENT (PAGE 163)

Mark Johnson

Mark Johnson is a Qigong (Chi Kung) healer and Qigong/T'ai Ji instructor in three styles. He also teaches Feng Shui, I Ching, and Chinese calligraphy, and studied with several famous Taoist masters in the USA, China and Taiwan. He has taught for over 30 years and officiated at over 50 T'ai Ji tournaments. Mark is a Founding Board Member of the National Qigong (Chi Kung) Association * USA, and has sold over 500,000 videos: *Tai Chi for Healing*, *Tai Chi for Women*, and *Tai Chi for Seniors*.

30 Elaine Ave., Mill Valley, CA 94941, USA

Tel/Fax: 1-800-497-4244
E-mail: chigung@mindspring.com
Web site: www.chi-kung.com

BABIES AND CHILDREN (PAGE 169)

Damaris Jarboux
(See Chi Kung Healing *above*)

Gaspar García

(See Buddhist Chi Kung *above*)

CHI KUNG AND THE ELDERLY (PAGE 174)

Tina Marrow Rasheed

As a certified health educator in Atlanta, Georgia, Tina applies her knowledge and experience of Qi Gong in the development and implementation of health promotion and disease prevention programs. Tina is committed to providing education and service to those most in need—medically underserved and senior populations. She also directs SelfWorks, a non-profit organization focused on assisting in the identification and management of stressors in everyday life.

630 Atlanta Avenue, Suite 2B,   Tel: 404-622-4259
Atlanta, GA 30312, USA   E-mail: marrowc@aol.com

CHI KUNG FOR SPECIAL NEEDS (PAGE 178)

Linda Chase Broda

Linda Broda has been teaching Tai Chi and Chi Kung for 20 years, at her own school in Manchester, UK, and throughout Europe. She has worked in hospitals and health centers, and with people with special needs. She is the Founding Chairperson of the Tai Chi and Chi Kung Forum for Health and Special Needs which trains teachers. Linda has produced a video of her work, *Tai Chi and Special Needs*, and written numerous articles for magazines.

Village Hall Tai Chi,   Tel: 0161-445-1568
163 Palatine Road, Manchester M20 2GH, Fax: 0161-445-9568
UK   E-mail: lindachasebroda@compuserve.com
                                       Web site: www.taichiandspecialneeds.co.uk

196 DEVELOPING YOUR ENERGY WITH PARTNERS AND GROUPS (PAGE 180)

Ronnie Robinson

Ronnie Robinson has studied Taijiquan and Qigong since 1981. He is editor of *Tai Chi Chuan and Internal Arts* magazine, Secretary of the Tai Chi Union for Great Britain, and Secretary of the Taijiquan and Qigong Federation for Europe. He teaches a variety of programs and classes in Scotland, and produces annual Wholistic Health and Natural Healing Festivals and Conferences.

Chiron Taijiquan & Qigong,
(Secretary-TCUGB),
1 Littlemill Drive, Balmoral Gardens,
Crookston, Glasgow, G53 7GF, UK

Tel: 0141-810-3482
Fax: 0141 810 3741
E-mail: chiron@dial.pipex.com

CHI KUNG—HEALING FOR THE WORLD (PAGE 182)

Bill Douglas

Bill Douglas is author of the #1 best selling T'ai Chi book, *The Complete Idiot's Guide to T'ai Chi & Qigong* (Alpha 2002, 2nd Edition), *The Amateur Parent* (SMART Prod. 2002), and *The Miracle of Stress*. Bill is a Founder of World T'ai Chi & Qigong Day.

Contact www.worldtaichiday.org to get involved with World T'ai Chi and Qigong Day. To order Bill's acclaimed video/audio series, contact www.smartaichi.com

Useful Addresses

EUROPE

The Taijiquan and Qigong Federation for Europe,
1 Littlemill Drive, Balmoral Gardens,
Crookston, Glasgow G53 7GF, UK

Tel: 0141-810-3482
Fax: 0141-810-3741
E-mail: info@tcfe.org
Web site: www.tcfe.org

The European Luohan Gong Federation,
Paseo de Colombia 172 A, Elviria,
Marbella 29600, Málaga, Spain

Tel: 34-95-283-4471
Fax: 34-95-276-4305
E-mail: gaspargarcia@salusline.com
Web sites: www.luohan.com and
www.salusline.com

The Tai Chi & Qigong Union for Great Britain,
1 Littlemill Drive, Balmoral Gardens,
Crookston, Glasgow G53 7GF, UK

Tel: 0141-810-3482
Fax: 0141-810-3741
E-mail: secretary@taichiunion.com
Web site: www.taichiunion.com

The Chi Kung School,
Great Georges Community Cultural Project
(The Blackie),
Great George Street, Liverpool L1 5EW, UK

Tel: 0151-709-5109
Fax: 0151-709-4822
Email: billharpe@theblackie.org.uk

Authentic Movement,
Larry Butler,
14 Garrioch Drive,
Glasgow, G20 8RS
Scotland, UK

Tel: 0141-946-8096
Web site: butlerlarry@hotmail.com

USA

National Qigong (Chi Kung) Association * USA,
PO Box 540, Ely, MN 55731, USA

Tel: 218-365-6330
Fax: 218-365-6933
E-mail: info@nqa.org
Web site: www.nqa.org

The Chi Kung School at The Body-Energy Center,

2730 29th St., Boulder, CO 80301, USA

Tel: 303-442-3131
Fax: 303-442-3141
Email: jamesmacritchie@earthlink.net
Web site: www.thebodyenergycenter.com

Healing Tao USA,

PO Box 601, Asheville, NC 28802, USA

Tel/Fax: 973-777-4442 and 888-999-0555
Email: info@HealingTaoUSA.com
Web site: www.HealingTaoUSA.com

Qigong Association of America,

2021 NW Grant Ave.,
Corvallis, OR 97330, USA

Tel: 541-752-6599
E-mail: dean@qi.org
Web site: www.qi.org

B.K. Frantzis,

Energy Arts, Inc., P.O. Box 99,
Fairfax, CA 94978, USA

Tel: 415-454-5243
Fax: 415-454-0907
E-mail: energyarts@energyarts.com
Web site: www.energyarts.com

The Anna Wise Center—Awakened Mind Training,

1000A Magnolia Ave., Larkspur, CA 94939, USA

Tel: 415-925-9449
E-mail: annawise2000@cs.com
Web site: www.annawise.com

The Empty Vessel—A Journal of Contemporary Taoism,

1991 Garfield St., Eugene, OR 97405, USA

Tel/Fax: 541-345-8854
E-mail: solala@abodetao.com
Web site: www.abodetao.com

Qi—The Journal of Traditional Eastern Health & Fitness (Qi Journal)

PO Box 18476, Anaheim Hills, CA 92817, USA

Tel: 714-779-1796
Fax: 714-779-1798
E-mail: editor@qi-journal.com
Web site: www.qi-journal.com

WORLDWIDE

The World Academic Society of Medical Qigong,

11 Bei San Huan Dong Rd.,
Chaoyang District, Beijing 100029, China

Tel: 86-(0)10-64286908
Fax: 86-(0)10-64211591

Glossary

Acupoints—energy points on the surface of the body.

Acupuncture—the insertion of hair-fine needles and the burning of a plant leaf called moxa on acupoints to affect the meridian energy. There are many different forms and styles of Acupuncture, such as Classical, Traditional, Symptomatic Formula, and Electro.

Adept—same as Master.

Aura field—the energy cocoon that projects out from and surrounds the physical body.

Ayurvedic—East Indian system of medicine.

Bioenergetics—a recently developed Western method of working with energy in the body and its relationship to psychotherapy: derived from the work of Wilhelm Reich.

Body-energy—all forms and aspects of energy in the body.

Cauldrons—major energy centers along the Thrusting channel/Chong Mo.

Chakras—energy centers within the body, as Cauldrons.

Chi—your energy for life.

Chi Kung Healer—a person who uses Chi Kung to heal.

Cultural Body-Energy Models—body-energy systems that have developed in a total cultural context.

Dao Yin/Tu Na/Tugu Naxin—older names for what is now known as Chi Kung.

Dynamic Meditation—a style of meditation that encourages the body to make spontaneous movement.

Dynamic/External/Wei Dan—postures and movements of Chi Kung.

Eight Principles—a way of describing energy in terms of its basic polarities: Yin/Yang, interior/exterior, excessive/deficient, hot/cold.

Electromagnetic spectrum—the spectrum of electromagnetic energy as defined by contemporary Western science.

Energy Body—the total of all of the body-energy systems, especially extending out beyond the physical body.

Fa Jing—energy projected out of the body by a Chi Kung healer.

Gross anatomy—the material substance of the physical body.

Hsien—a realized and enlightened person.

I Ching—The Book of Changes.

Immortality—the continuation of the soul/spirit after physical death.

Impersonal, Transpersonal—beyond the individual ego identity, and relating to the higher self.

Inner Alchemy—the spiritual tradition and training.

Jing—the primary energy inherited from your ancestors, and the basis of sexual energy.

Kundalini—a refined energy that ascends the spine in Yoga.

Kung—cultivating, developing, working with.

Laokung— point on the palms; also called "Palace of Weariness."

Master—a person who has been conferred this title by their Teacher/Master, showing that they have reached the highest levels of achievement in a particular practice.

Medical Chi Kung—the application of Chi Kung by a healer for medical reasons.

Meridian system—the pathway of 35 energy lines according to the Oriental tradition, including the twelve organ meridians, the eight extra meridians, and the related subsidiary pathways.

Metaphorical and Symbolic language—non-descriptive language understandable only to the initiated, usually intended to protect the meaning of a statement.

Microcosmic Orbit: Small Heaven Circuit—the circulation of energy along the Governor and Conception meridians.

Mingmen—point on the center line of the back, between the second and third lumbar vertebrae; also called "Gate of Life."

Mo—Meridian/Channel/Vessel, Energy pathway.

Nadis—a network of energy lines in the Yoga system.

Nei Ching—Huang Ti Nei Ching—The Yellow Emperor's Classic of Internal Medicine.

Nurse healer—a nurse who practices Therapeutic Touch and hands-on healing.

Organs/Officials—the 12 primary organs and functions.

Pa Kua—the Buddhist eight-sided figure/octagon, each side containing a trigram.

Paihui—point on the crown of the head; also called "One Hundred Meetings."

Pulses—six points on each wrist that inform a practitioner about the state and condition of the 12 major organs/officials.

Qi Gong, Qigong, Chi Gung—alternative spellings of Chi Kung.

Quiescent Chi Kung—preparatory practice to calm and clear oneself.

Shaman—a priest or practitioner who can control and influence events in both the material and spirit worlds.

Shaolin—a temple famous for its martial arts and Chi Kung.

Shen—the spirit.

Sifu—Teacher.

Sole cultivation and dual cultivation—sexual practice to preserve the Jing.

Static/Internal/Nei Dan—meditation and mental control of Chi Kung.

Subtle anatomy/Energy anatomy—the structure of the energy system.

Ta Chi/Ku Chi/Wei Chi/Yuan Chi/Ching Chi/Hsien-T'ien Chi/Jing Chi—terms for various manifestations of internal energy in the body.

Table of Correspondence—the correlations of things and qualities assigned to each of the Five Elements.

T'ai Chi Chuan—a movement form used for martial arts or health conditioning, of which there are numerous variations and schools.

Tao Te Ching—the first classic of Taoism, said to be written by the sage Lao Tzu.

Taoism—the philosophy/religion espousing The Tao, as expounded by Lao Tzu.

Traditional Chinese Medicine (TCM) —the title given by the Communist Government in The
People's Republic of China to describe their comprehensive system of medicine, including acupuncture and herbalism.

The Eight Extraordinary Meridians—the meridians that function as reservoirs of energy, comprising Governor (Du Mo), Conception (Ren Mo), Thrusting (Chong Mo), Girdle (Dai Mo), Arm and Leg Linking and Connecting (Yang Qiao Mo, Yin Qiao Mo, Yang Wei Mo, Yin Wei Mo).

The Eight Immortals—the saints of folk Taoism.

The Five Elements—a system for classifying nature in terms of its essential characteristics—Wood, Fire, Earth, Metal, and Water.

The Pearl—the condensed essence of body-energy into a small ball.

The Tao—The Way of Nature.

Therapeutic Touch—a contemporary Western title for a process that uses the hands as a focus to facilitate healing; the Western equivalent of Medical Chi Kung and Chi Kung Healing.

Three Chou—the areas of the upper, middle, and lower abdomen.

Three Heater/Triple Heater—one of the 12 meridians/officials which controls temperature, amongst other functions.

Three Tan T'ien/Three Elixir Fields/Three Fields of Cultivation—centers of energy in the lower abdomen, mid-torso, and head.

Three Treasures—Jing, Chi, and Shen.

Twelve Organ Meridians—the part of the meridian system related to each of the 12 major organs/officials.

Wei Chi—external healing

Wu Wei—non-action, non-interference, the path of least resistance.

Yang Jing—Male primary, sexual energy.

Yin/Yang—the primary polarity of natural phenomena.

Yin Jing—Female primary, sexual energy.

Yin Tang—Original Cavity of the pure spirit.

Yungchuan—point on the soles of the feet; also called "Bubbling Spring."

Further Reading

BOOKS BY JAMES MACRITCHIE

The State of Play—Theatre Games as Social Art, (with Bill Harpe), Great Georges Community Arts Project, 1972

Exit to Enter: Dance As A Process Of Personal And Artistic Growth, (with Anna Halprin), San Francisco Dancers Workshop, 1973

Chi Kung: Cultivating Personal Energy, Element Books, 1993

The Chi Kung Way—Alive with Energy, HarperCollins, 1997

The Chinese Way To Health, (Chi Kung section in book by Dr. Stephen Gascoigne M.D.), Charles Tuttle & Co., 1997

CHI KUNG/QIGONG

Mantak and Maneewan Chia et al., *Awakening Healing Light—Tao Energetic Medicine Of The Future,* Healing Tao Books, 1993

— *Taoist Secrets Of Love—Cultivating Male Sexual Energy,* Aurora Press, 1984

— *Healing Love Through The Tao—Cultivating Female Sexual Energy,* Healing Tao Books, 1986

— *Chi Nei Tsang—Internal Organ Chi Massage,* Healing Tao Books, 1992

Effie Poy Yew Chow, *Miracle Healing From China,* Medipress, 1996

Bill Douglas, *The Complete Idiot's Guide to T'ai Chi and Qigong,* MacMillan, 1998

John Du Cane, *The Five Animal Frolics,* Dragon Door, 1999

Francesco Garri Garripoli, *Qigong—Essence of the Healing Dance,* Health Communications Inc., 1999

B.K. Frantzis, *Opening The Energy Gates Of Your Body,* North Atlantic Books, 1993

— *The Power of Internal Martial Arts,* North Atlantic Books, 1998

— (The Water Method of Taoist Meditation Series), *Volume 1, Relaxing Into Your Being,* Clarity Press, 1998

— (The Water Method of Taoist Meditation Series), *Volume 2, The Great Stillness,* Clarity Press, 1999

Roger Jahnke, *The Healer Within,* HarperSanFrancisco, 1997

— *The Most Profound Medicine,* Health Action Publishing, 1988

— *The Self-Applied Health Enhancement Methods,* Health Action Publishing, 1989

— *The Healing Promise of Qi,* Contemporary Books, 2002

Jerry Alan Johnson, *Chinese Medical Qigong Therapy: A Comprehensive Clinical Text,* The International Institute of Medical Qigong, 2000

Yanling Johnson, *A Women's Qigong Guide,* YMAA, 2001

— *Qi & You,* YMAA Pub. Co., 2002

Dennis Lewis, *The Tao Of Natural Breathing,* Mountain Wind Publishing, 1997

Adrian Lowe, *The Art of Daoyin,* Lamas Qigong Association, 1998

Daniel P. Reid, *Harnessing The Power Of The Universe,* Shambhala, 1998

The I Ching or Book of Changes, (Richard Wilhelm, trans.), Princeton University Press, 1950

Tao Te Ching, (Stephen Mitchell, trans.), HarperCollins, 1988

John Blofeld, *Taoism—The Road to Immortality*, Shambhala, 2000

Thomas Cleary, *The Inner Teachings Of Taoism*, Shambhala, 1986

— *Understanding Reality*, University Of Hawaii Press, 1987

— *Immortal Sisters—Secrets Of Taoist Women*, Shambhala, 1989

James Legge, *The I Ching—The Book Of Changes*, Dover Publications, 1963

K'uan Yu Lu (Charles Luk), *The Secrets Of Chinese Meditation*, Samuel Weiser, 1984

Thomas Merton, *The Way of Chuang Tzu*, New Directions Paperbook, 1969

Hua Ching Ni, *The Book of Changes and the Unchanging Truth*, The Shrine of the Eternal Breath of Tao, 1983

Solala Towler, *A Gathering Of Cranes: Bringing The Tao to the West*, Abode of the Eternal Tao Pub. Co., 1997

— *Embarking on the Way: A Guide to Western Taoism*, Abode of the Eternal Tao Pub. Co., 1998

Burton Watson, *Chuang Tzu—Basic Writings*, Columbia University Press, 1964

Richard Wilhelm, *The Secret Of The Golden Flower*, Harcourt Brace Jovanovich, 1962

Eva Wong, *Seven Taoist Masters*, Shambhala, 1990

— *Cultivating Stillness*, Shambala, 1992

RELATED SOURCES

Harriet Beinfield and Efrem Korngold, *Between Heaven and Earth*, Ballantine Books, 1991

Dan Bensky and John O'Connor, *Acupuncture—A Comprehensive Text*, Eastland Press, 1981

Joseph Needham, *Science and Civilisation in China*, Cambridge University Press, 1954

Maoshing Ni, *The Yellow Emperor's Classic of Medicine*, Shambhala, 1995

David Scott and Tony Doubleday, *The Elements of Zen*, Element Books, 1992

Katya Walter, *The Tao Of Chaos*, Kairos Center, 1994

Anna Wise, *The High Performance Mind*, Tarcher/Putnam, 1995

— *Awakening the Mind. A Guide to Mastering the Power of your Brainwaves*, Tarcher/Putnam, 2002

J.R. Worsley, *Traditional Chinese Acupuncture—Vol. I. Meridians and Points*, Element Books, The College Of Traditional Chinese Acupuncture, UK, 1982

— *Traditional Acupuncture—Vol. II. Traditional Diagnosis*, The College of Traditional Chinese Acupuncture, UK, 1990

— *Traditional Acupuncture Vol III. The Five Elements—The Officials*, The College of Traditional Chinese Medicine, 1996

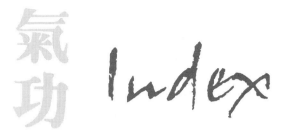

Index